# INTERMITTENT FASTING FOR WOMEN OVER 50 SIMPLIFIED

Your Path to Hormonal Balance, Healthy Weight
Management, and Increased Energy Without the
Hassle

RADIANTSHE

# Contents

# Introduction

Imagine this: You're seated at the dining table, alone with your thoughts, staring at a plate of grilled chicken and steamed vegetables. It's a familiar scene that often prompts reflections on the changes life throws our way after reaching the half-century mark. You wonder, "Is this the peak of aging, or is there a better way?"

Navigating life as a woman over 50 can feel like walking a tightrope, with each step bringing its challenges. Hormonal imbalances, once distant concerns, now take center stage as we approach menopause. Mood swings, hot flashes, and night sweats become our new reality, disrupting not just our physical well-being but also our emotional and mental health. Weight management becomes an uphill battle as our metabolism begins to slow down. The dieting methods that once yielded results now seem futile, leaving us frustrated and defeated. The struggle to find sustainable weight loss strategies that align with our changing bodies and lifestyles becomes all-consuming as we long for control over our health and well-being.

Each day, our energy levels seem to dwindle, leaving us drained. Activities that once brought us joy now feel like daunting tasks as we struggle to keep up with the demands of daily life. The desire to regain our youthful vitality becomes a constant companion, driving us to seek methods to boost our energy levels and reclaim our zest for life. Navigating the maze of online nutritional advice adds to our confusion and frustration. The barrage of conflicting information leaves us wanting to figure out where to turn. What should we eat? When should we eat? How does fasting fit into the equation? These questions loom large in our minds, fueling our quest for precise, reliable guidance that speaks to our age and unique dietary needs.

If you've also found yourself feeling like this, then you're not alone. Statistics paint a stark picture of the challenges women over 50 encounter. Around 75% of women experience menopausal symptoms like hot flashes and mood swings. Moreover, over 43% of women battle with menopausal obesity, highlighting the struggle many face in maintaining a healthy weight. And with over 80% of Americans admitting to feeling confused by conflicting nutritional information, it's no wonder that making the right food choices can feel like an uphill battle. 70% of menopausal women experience increased emotional states like anger and anxiety, decreased concentration, and decreased confidence and self-esteem.

While the journey past 50 brings its own set of challenges, It's a reality many women face, but it's not one you must navigate

alone. For many women over 50, seeking out a book like this isn't just a casual choice—it's a necessity born out of a deeply felt need for change. Emotionally, you may grapple with frustration, disillusionment, and even a sense of loss. Sense of imbalance that disrupts their daily lives and relationships. Physically, you may be contending with the challenges of weight gain, fatigue, and aches and pains that seem to accompany aging.

Amidst these challenges, the decision to pick up this book is a beacon of hope—a declaration of your commitment to reclaiming their health, vitality, and well-being. You are searching for practical solutions, reliable guidance, and a sense of community to support them on their journey towards a better, brighter future. This book is a lifeline, offering the promise of transformation and renewal you crave.

Enter the VIBRANT method – your roadmap to success. Each letter represents a crucial aspect of intermittent fasting tailored specifically for women over 50:

- **V** - Vision for Intermittent Fasting: Set clear goals and envision the outcomes you desire from your intermittent fasting journey.
- **I** - Introduction to Hormonal Health: Understand how hormonal changes impact your body and learn personalized solutions to manage symptoms effectively.

- **B** - Balanced Recipes and Meal Plans: Discover delicious and nutritious recipes to support your intermittent fasting lifestyle.
- **R** - Routines in Exercise: Access safe and effective exercise routines tailored for older women, prioritizing safety and efficacy.
- **A** - Advanced Fasting Methods: Explore advanced fasting techniques to accelerate your results and enhance your fasting experience.
- **N** - Navigating Challenges: Learn how to overcome common obstacles and setbacks on your intermittent fasting journey.
- **T** - Transforming Your Life: Experience the transformative power of intermittent fasting as you regain control of your health and well-being.

By embracing intermittent fasting, you stand to gain tangible benefits:

- **Personalized Solutions for Hormonal Imbalance**: Gain insights into managing menopausal symptoms like hot flashes and mood swings.
- **Sustainable Weight Loss Strategies:** Say goodbye to fad diets and hello to lasting weight loss results tailored for your body.
- **Reclaim Your Energy:** Feel energized and revitalized as you implement lifestyle changes to support your well-being.
- **Clear Nutritional Guidance:** Eliminate nutrition confusion and make informed choices to fuel your body effectively.

- **Safe and Effective Fitness Tips:** Stay active with exercise routines designed specifically for older women, prioritizing safety and efficacy.

If you're wondering whether intermittent fasting works for women over 50, look no further than the countless success stories shared by women like you. From everyday individuals to celebrities, the evidence is clear: intermittent fasting can transform lives.

- Female, age 51- I began intermittent fasting for the first time this year on the 8:16 schedule on weekdays and 10:14 on weekends. I drink loads of natural teas. Nevertheless, I track my food variety in a diary (attempting to remain between 1,200 and 1,500 daily). I have shed right around 10 pounds this month! This is, by all accounts, working for me.
- Female, 53- "I started 16:8 a little over a year ago. I'm not super-strict with my calories and carbs, but I am down around 27 lbs since I began."
- Female,50- "16:8 after two months, 15 lbs down. I didn't think this was possible at my age, but it is!"
- Female, 68 -"I've been doing IF for 12 years. I lost 60 lbs and have kept it off by doing 20/4. I was a compulsive overeater all my life- binge eating- and tried everything to get my weight under control. IF is the only thing that worked, taking away the compulsion to eat constantly, and I only wish I'd found it 40 years earlier!!!"

A better life is possible for us all, even if it might not feel like it now. So, as you embark on this journey, know that you've made the right choice. You're not just reading a book – you're joining a community of women committed to reclaiming their vitality and embracing the best years of their lives. Together, let's unlock the power of intermittent fasting and embark on a journey to renewed health and well-being.

ONE

# Vision for Intermittent Fasting

> "To eat when you are sick is to feed your sickness."

Hippocrates

Welcome to the beginning of your journey toward renewed vitality and well-being. As you embark on this chapter, imagine a world where your body feels energized, your hormones are in harmony, and your weight is managed effortlessly. Intermittent Fasting offers a pathway to this reality. In the pages ahead, we'll explore why it's not just a fad but a lifestyle shift with profound implications, especially for women over 50.

## What Is Intermittent Fasting?

Intermittent Fasting ( IF) involves cycling between periods of eating and Fasting, with the primary focus on when you eat rather than what you eat. While there are various methods of intermittent Fasting, ranging from the 16/8 method to alternate-day Fasting, the underlying principle remains the same: giving your body extended periods of rest from digestion to facilitate various physiological processes.

So why has intermittent Fasting gained traction recently, particularly among older adults? The answer lies in its potential to address some of the unique challenges faced by individuals in this demographic, from hormonal imbalances to metabolic slowdown. But before we delve into its benefits for women over 50, let's take a step back and explore its historical and cultural roots.

## The History of Fasting

Fasting has been practiced for centuries across different cultures and civilizations. Religious Fasting was widespread in various ancient civilizations, spanning countries such as India, China, the Middle East, and Greece. Religions stood and developed their fasting rituals to support their spiritual development. Some, for example, regarded intermittent Fasting as a way of purifying the soul and drawing oneself nearer to spiritual rewards, such as forging a closer connection with the divine. This purpose endures today, ingrained within various modern cultures and religions.

Ancient civilizations, from the Greeks to the Egyptians, recognized the therapeutic benefits of Fasting and utilized it to treat various ailments.

In recent history, Fasting has been a cornerstone of medical practices such as Ayurveda and Traditional Chinese Medicine, which was employed to cleanse the body, promote longevity, and restore balance. Today, intermittent Fasting represents a modern adaptation of these ancient practices, harnessing the body's innate ability to heal and regenerate.

Interest in intermittent Fasting has surged in recent years thanks to scientific research and media coverage. However, delving into its origins reveals a profound truth: intermittent Fasting has a rich and enduring history that stretches back centuries. As we explore its roots, we uncover a tapestry woven by diverse civilizations and ancient healers who recognized the importance of aligning our eating patterns with the natural rhythms of life. This historical perspective adds depth and context to our modern understanding of intermittent Fasting, highlighting its timeless relevance and the wisdom of those who came before us.

Intermittent Fasting is a resurgence of ancient knowledge, a return to the intuitive insight that our bodies, like the seasons, flourish in cycles. It is not a transitory fad but rather a continuum—a link between historical knowledge and current goals. Historical fasting traditions demonstrate a widespread understanding of its benefits for spiritual, physical, and therapeutic objectives.

Let us explore the processes of Fasting, including the phases and scientific foundations that connect them. Unraveling the complexity of this biological and physiological phenomenon is critical for demystifying its effectiveness, and we certainly want you to begin your fast with solid knowledge.

## The Science Behind Fasting

At its core, intermittent Fasting triggers biological and physiological responses that promote health and longevity. From metabolic shifts to cellular repair mechanisms, fasting engages the body's natural resilience and adaptability. Intermittent Fasting triggers a series of intricate biological and physiological processes in women, which can be understood through various stages of Fasting. During the initial fasting phase, typically within the first 12 to 24 hours, the body exhausts its immediate glycogen stores for energy. This depletion prompts a shift in metabolism, leading to the breakdown of stored fat into fatty acids and glycerol to fuel cellular function.

As Fasting continues beyond 24 hours into the early stages of the fast, the body enters a state of ketosis. Ketosis occurs when the liver converts fatty acids into ketone bodies, which serve as an alternative fuel source for tissues and organs, particularly the brain. This metabolic switch enhances cognitive function and mental clarity while preserving lean muscle mass.

In the intermediate stages of Fasting, typically beyond 48 hours, the body undergoes autophagy—a cellular cleansing process. During autophagy, damaged or dysfunctional cellular components are broken down and recycled, promoting cellular renewal and rejuvenation. This process is crucial in reducing inflammation, enhancing cellular repair, and bolstering immune function.

One essential process that occurs during Fasting is autophagy. This cellular cleaning process removes damaged or dysfunctional components and promotes cellular renewal. By clearing out cellular debris, autophagy plays a crucial role in maintaining cellular health and function, with implications for aging and disease prevention.

Moreover, recent scientific investigations have unearthed a plethora of evidence affirming the effectiveness of intermittent Fasting across various health domains, encompassing weight management, metabolic well-being, and cognitive prowess. Research indicates intermittent Fasting can bolster metabolic adaptability, enhance insulin sensitivity, and foster cognitive acuity. Even without significant weight loss, adjusting meal timings, such as advancing breakfast and elongating the overnight fasting period, has demonstrated considerable metabolic benefits (Harvard et al., 2021).

The authors elucidate that intermittent Fasting's enduring benefits stem from its capacity to elicit lasting adaptive responses upon repeated exposure to fasting intervals. These "broad-spectrum benefits" not only confer resilience against various diseases but also augment mental and physical performance (National Institute of Aging, 2020).

A study involving 23 obese participants investigated the repercussions of restricting eating to a specific window, from 10 a.m. to 6 p.m., over 12 weeks. During this timeframe, participants had unrestricted food choices within the designated hours. On average, participants consumed approximately 350 fewer calories, experienced a modest 3% reduction in body weight, and observed a decline in systolic blood pressure (UIC Today, 2021).

## Benefits of Intermittent Fasting for Women Over 50

Now, let's focus on the specific benefits of intermittent Fasting for women in your age group. Hormonal balance, weight management, and increased energy levels are just a few of the potential advantages that intermittent Fasting can offer.

- **Hormonal Balance:** For women navigating menopause and hormonal changes, intermittent Fasting can be crucial in restoring hormonal balance. Research suggests Fasting can regulate hormone levels, including insulin, growth hormone, and cortisol, which are essential for metabolic health and overall well-being. By promoting hormonal equilibrium, intermittent Fasting may alleviate symptoms such as hot flashes, mood swings, and sleep disturbances, enhancing the quality of life during this transitional phase.

- **Weight Loss:** Many women over 50 struggle with weight management due to age-related metabolic changes and hormonal fluctuations. Intermittent Fasting offers a promising solution by promoting fat loss while preserving lean muscle mass. By restricting the eating window or incorporating fasting days, individuals can create a calorie deficit, leading to weight loss over time. Additionally, intermittent Fasting enhances metabolic flexibility, improves insulin sensitivity, and boosts fat oxidation, making it a powerful tool for sustainable weight management in older women.

- **Increased Energy Levels:** As women age, declining energy levels can impact daily functioning and overall vitality. Intermittent Fasting has been shown to enhance energy levels by optimizing metabolic function and promoting cellular regeneration. By utilizing stored fat for fuel during fasting periods, the body can maintain steady energy levels throughout the day, reducing fatigue and enhancing mental clarity. Many women report feeling more energized and focused after incorporating intermittent Fasting into their routine, allowing them to stay active and engaged in various activities.

However, that is not all. Intermittent Fasting has been shown to have a broad spectrum of health benefits. For example, Intermittent Fasting has emerged as a potential promoter of thyroid hormone output, which is crucial for maintaining optimal bone health. By fostering a hormonal environment conducive to balance, intermittent Fasting may aid in preventing conditions like osteoporosis, arthritis, and lower back pain. This hormonal aspect of Fasting could be pivotal in enhancing bone density and resilience, offering a comprehensive approach to musculoskeletal well-being. In essence, intermittent Fasting may fortify bones and reduce the risk of fractures.

Moreover, as we delve into the manifold benefits of intermittent Fasting, it becomes evident that it profoundly impacts brain health. Research indicates fasting shields brain neurons from degeneration and dysfunction (Philips, 2019), thereby preserving and enhancing cognitive function. Recent studies released in 2021 further bolster this notion, suggesting that Fasting might maintain and potentially improve memory and defend against neurological ailments like Alzheimer's disease and strokes (Lawler, 2019). These cognitive advantages underscore another facet of intermittent Fasting's positive influence on overall health.

Furthermore, intermittent Fasting extends its benefits beyond physical health to mental and emotional well-being. It shows promise in alleviating anxiety, depression, stress, and emotional fluctuations associated with hormonal changes and aging while also boosting self-esteem and vitality. This recognition of the intricate interplay between dietary choices, mental health, and life perspectives underscores intermittent Fasting's holistic approach to our well-being.

Additionally, intermittent Fasting may contribute to better-quality sleep at night. Although the precise mechanisms are not fully understood, hypotheses suggest that intermittent Fasting may influence sleep patterns by regulating the circadian rhythm, simplifying falling asleep, and promoting a feeling of refreshment upon waking. Another theory posits that fasting on an empty stomach may reduce heartburn and digestion-related disturbances, improving sleep quality (Lawler, 2019).

## Separating Myths from Facts

Before we conclude this chapter, we must address some common misconceptions surrounding intermittent Fasting. Despite its growing popularity, intermittent Fasting is often misunderstood and misrepresented. From concerns about nutrient deficiencies to fears of metabolic damage, these myths can deter individuals from exploring intermittent Fasting as a viable lifestyle option.

**Myth—Fasting means starving myself**

**Fact:** It's essential to emphasize that intermittent Fasting is not synonymous with starvation. Unlike starvation, where the body lacks vital nutrients for prolonged periods, intermittent Fasting involves strategic periods of eating and Fasting, allowing the body to receive necessary nutrients during feeding windows. Additionally, most intermittent fasting protocols do not restrict overall calorie intake but instead regulate the timing of meals, making it unlikely to lead to severe nutrient deficiencies when followed appropriately.

**Myth—Fasting slows metabolism**

**Fact**—Dispelling the myth that Fasting wreaks havoc on your metabolic processes, recent research suggests a more rejuvenating narrative—it may well breathe fresh life into metabolic activities if the advantages it provides to your system have not convinced you. Fasting causes an increase in metabolic regulators such as norepinephrine and other growth hormones. This upswing allows your body to navigate the terrain of accessible fuel sources with ease. According to a study by Zhang et al. in 2023, there is a risk of metabolic health problems and an increased susceptibility to illness. Surprisingly, this research shows that fasting for up to 48 hours might result in a metabolic increase ranging from 3.6% to 14%. Though this might seem excessive, research also supports short durations of fasting, claiming that "short-term fasts may increase your metabolic rate" (Gunnars, 2019). So, a metabolic halt? A myth.

**Myth—Fasting causes muscle loss**

**Fact**—Muscles are essential to our general health and are sometimes called the organ of longevity. Maintaining proper muscular mass, particularly skeletal muscles, provides metabolic advantages and improves well-being. Unfortunately, aging is associated with muscle loss, leading to various health issues. The idea that Fasting may exacerbate this problem is prevalent, but research provides a reassuring viewpoint. Studies have shown that Fasting retains lean muscle mass and even increases muscular development (Laurens et al., 2021). Fasting causes the release of growth hormones and metabolic changes, which promote muscle development, preservation, and protein conservation. It is critical to eliminate the myth that fasting results in nutritional shortage. Even when fasting, ingesting protein and nutrient-dense meals is essential to providing the body with the required building blocks. When done appropriately, Fasting can have the opposite impact, improving muscular health and metabolic well-being.

**Myth—Fasting is not safe**

**Fact**—Fasting is sometimes stigmatized as unhealthy due to worries about dehydration, hunger, and disturbances in basic functioning. Contrary to popular belief, Fasting is entirely safe when done correctly and can provide several advantages.

Problems develop when people need to make better dietary choices or follow fasting recommendations, such as missing water, overindulging in harmful foods during the eating window, or ignoring critical nutrients.

Numerous studies have proven the relationship between Fasting and various health advantages, with some proposing that it may lead to "a longer and all-around healthier life" (Gunnars, 2021).

**Myth—Fasting is only about losing weight**

Fact—While Fasting is an excellent approach for weight loss, it goes beyond the restricted objective of losing pounds temporarily. It differs from other diets geared for short-term weight loss by stressing a holistic approach to health. The fundamental concept of Fasting is well-being, and the attendant health advantages automatically follow. Weight loss may be a result if linked with personal goals. Overall, the goal is to promote long-term health and vitality.

**Myth—Fasting has no scientific proof**

Fact—While the notion persists that insufficient data supports the advantages of Fasting, the truth is precisely the opposite. Numerous studies have conclusively established the benefits of fasting in various health categories, including weight loss, cardiovascular health, and cognitive performance. Mark Mattson, a prominent investigator at the National Institute on Aging, claims that Fasting has consistently improved disease biomarkers, decreased oxidative stress, and preserved learning and memory abilities (Collier, 2013). Furthermore, in 2022, Johns Hopkins Medicine published an article compiling a collection of studies supporting the benefits of Fasting, such as its capacity to improve verbal memory in adults. The range of studies validates the favorable effects of Fasting.

**Myth—All Intermittent Fasting is the same**

**Fact**—Navigating the world of intermittent Fasting offers a plethora of regimens, each defined by distinct eating windows and fasting intervals. The key to successfully practicing Fasting is to link the selected approach with specific health and fitness objectives. Clearly outlining these objectives is critical since it directs the selection of the fasting type that best achieves your intended results. It is equally important to consider long-term sustainability while implementing a fasting habit. The efficacy of Fasting is dependent on its flawless integration into your current lifestyle, reducing disturbances and creating a harmonic match. Fasting becomes a personalized method that empowers you as the orchestrator, allowing you to keep control while receiving the fundamental advantages.

**Myth—Fasting makes you overindulge and binge**

**Fact**--- is a lack of evidence for the myth that post-fasting eating always leads to overindulgence. For example, one research found that those who fasted for one day ingested only around 500 calories extra the next day, much less than the 2,400 calories they missed during their fast (Johnstone et al., 2002). The apparent inclination to overeat after Fasting may be due to the mind-game component of dieting. The mental discourse around constraints and ideas such as "I cannot eat right now" can alter your perception of food and drive you to overeat or binge. However, all of this is in the mind, and turning away from this crucial way of thinking.

As we wrap up this chapter, I invite you to reflect on the insights we have uncovered together. Intermittent Fasting is not just a dietary strategy but a journey toward holistic well-being and vitality. In the chapters ahead, we will continue to explore the transformative power of Intermittent Fasting and its profound implications for your health and happiness. So stay tuned, and let us embark on this journey together.

In the next chapter, we'll dive deeper into the topic of hormonal health and how Intermittent Fasting can help restore balance in your body. Hormonal health is especially critical for women over 50, and by understanding how Intermittent Fasting impacts hormones, you'll be better equipped to harness its full potential.

# TWO

# Introduction to Hormonal Health

> "Hormones are like tiny messengers in our bodies, sometimes delivering love, sometimes unleashing chaos."
>
> Unknown

Welcome to the intricate world of hormonal health, where these tiny messengers wield immense power over our bodies and minds. Nowhere is this more evident than in women over 50, where hormonal fluctuations can feel like a rollercoaster ride of emotions and physical changes. In this chapter, we delve into the importance of hormonal health, especially for women navigating the complexities of midlife and beyond.

For women over 50, hormonal balance is not just a matter of comfort—it's a key determinant of overall well-being. From managing menopausal symptoms to preserving bone density and mental clarity, hormones play a vital role in every aspect of health. Yet, achieving and maintaining hormonal equilibrium can be daunting, often leading to frustration and uncertainty.

Enter intermittent fasting, a holistic approach to health that extends beyond mere weight management. Emerging research suggests intermittent fasting may offer a promising solution for optimizing hormonal balance in women over 50. By strategically timing periods of eating and fasting, individuals can modulate hormone levels and promote greater harmony within the body.

This chapter will explore the relationship between intermittent fasting and hormonal health, examining how fasting protocols may influence critical hormones such as insulin, cortisol, and estrogen. By understanding the mechanisms behind intermittent fasting and its impact on hormonal balance, women over 50 can empower themselves to take control of their health and embrace the journey towards hormonal harmony.

## How Intermittent Fasting Helps in Hormonal Balance

Before we dive into the specifics of intermittent fasting, let's first unravel the complexity of hormones. Hormones are chemicals that coordinate different bodily functions by carrying messages through your blood to your organs, skin, muscles, and other tissues. Hormones play a pivotal role in regulating various bodily functions, from metabolism to mood, and maintaining their equilibrium is crucial for overall well-being. "Hormones are complex and powerful chemicals. If one or more of them goes out of whack, it can cause certain symptoms that make you feel like you're not in control of your body." (Cleveland Clinic, 2022)

For women over 50, maintaining hormonal balance becomes especially crucial as they navigate through menopause—a period marked by significant hormonal fluctuations. Menopause, typically occurring around the age of 50, heralds the end of reproductive capacity and brings about a decline in estrogen and progesterone levels. These hormonal changes can trigger a cascade of symptoms, including hot flashes, night sweats, mood swings, and irregular periods. Additionally, fluctuations in thyroid hormones, cortisol, and insulin further compound this demographic's challenges of hormonal imbalance.

Hormones also play a pivotal role in maintaining bone density, cardiovascular health, cognitive function, and emotional stability. Imbalances in estrogen and progesterone levels, for example, can increase the risk of osteoporosis and heart disease. At the same time, fluctuations in cortisol may contribute to stress-related conditions such as anxiety and depression.

Furthermore, hormonal imbalances can disrupt metabolic processes, leading to weight gain, insulin resistance, and other metabolic disorders. "Thyroid hormones act to regulate the body's metabolism or the rate it burns energy. Too few thyroid hormones can slow metabolism and result in weight gain." (Huizen, 2023) Insulin, a hormone produced by the pancreas, regulates blood sugar levels and plays a central role in metabolism. When insulin levels are dysregulated, as seen in conditions like insulin resistance, individuals become more susceptible to diabetes and obesity.

Estrogen, ghrelin, Leptin, and insulin are hormones that can be impacted by age and lifestyle factors. Estrogen is a group of sex hormones primarily responsible for the development and regulation of the female reproductive system. Beyond its reproductive functions, estrogen also influences bone health, cardiovascular health, cognitive function, and mood regulation. During menopause, estrogen levels decline significantly, leading to a variety of symptoms such as hot flashes, night sweats, vaginal dryness, and mood swings. These hormonal changes can increase the risk of osteoporosis, heart disease, and cognitive decline in postmenopausal women.

Insulin is a hormone produced by the pancreas to regulate blood sugar levels. When cells become resistant to insulin, they fail to respond adequately to its signals, leading to elevated blood sugar levels and, eventually, type 2 diabetes. Insulin sensitivity is crucial for overall metabolic health, as it influences glucose uptake by cells, fat storage, and energy expenditure. Ghrelin and Leptin are hormones involved in regulating appetite and energy balance. Ghrelin, often called the "hunger hormone," stimulates appetite and promotes food intake. In contrast, Leptin, known as the "satiety hormone," signals fullness and inhibits hunger. Imbalances in ghrelin and leptin levels can disrupt appetite regulation, leading to overeating, weight gain, and obesity.

But fear not, for intermittent fasting offers hope in the quest for hormonal harmony. Several studies have provided insights into how intermittent fasting affects vital hormones in metabolism, appetite regulation, and overall health. The article" The Link Between Fasting and Hormone Balance" (LifeMD,2023) highlights many of these benefits.

One significant effect is the reduction in insulin levels during fasting periods. The bloodstream experiences lower sugar levels with decreased food intake, prompting the pancreas to reduce insulin production. Consequently, the body shifts from utilizing glucose for energy to tapping into stored fat, facilitating fat breakdown and enhancing insulin sensitivity. This metabolic process not only aids in weight loss over time but also helps reduce oxidative stress, promoting better health outcomes. Additionally, leptin levels tend to decrease during fasting, especially in the initial stages of weight loss. This decline signals to the brain that the body's energy reserves are depleting, potentially triggering increased appetite and hunger sensations. However, as the body adapts to fasting periods, leptin levels stabilize, improving appetite control and reducing excessive eating.

Moreover, fasting impacts ghrelin levels, a hormone associated with hunger. While fasting initially increases ghrelin levels, prolonged fasting periods decrease ghrelin, contributing to enhanced appetite control. This reduction in ghrelin levels can be advantageous for individuals aiming to manage their calorie intake and lose weight effectively. Cortisol, another hormone affected by fasting, undergoes complex changes depending on the duration of fasting. Short-term fasting triggers increased cortisol levels as a natural response to stress and low blood sugar. However, extended fasting periods may cause cortisol levels to drop, potentially reducing the risk of stress-related health issues.

Furthermore, fasting has been observed to reduce excess body fat, which is often associated with elevated estrogen levels. As fat tissues can produce and store estrogen, decreasing body fat through fasting can help achieve a better hormonal balance, particularly for individuals with high estrogen levels associated with various health issues, including hormone-related cancer. Lastly, fasting can impact glucagon levels, stimulating the liver to release glucose to maintain stable blood sugar levels. This process ensures a continuous energy supply, primarily when the body utilizes stored fat for energy during fasting. The adjustment of glucagon levels also supports critical processes such as brain function, which rely on glucose for optimal performance.

## Alleviating Menopause Symptoms

Menopause is a natural transition in a woman's life, but it can also be a challenging one. At the heart of menopause are hormonal changes that can sometimes feel like a whirlwind of emotions and physical sensations. Your body, which once felt familiar, suddenly feels like it's speaking a different language. Hot flashes may come out of nowhere, leaving you feeling like you're standing in the middle of a desert on the hottest day of the year. Mood swings may turn you into a whirlwind of emotions, where laughter can quickly turn into tears without warning.

Menopause can trigger a variety of symptoms that can significantly impact a woman's quality of life. Many of these symptoms are tied to hormones. Among the most common are hot flashes, mood swings, and sleep disturbances, each of which is closely tied to fluctuations in hormone levels.

Hot flashes, also known as vasomotor symptoms, are perhaps one of the most notorious hallmarks of menopause. They can be described as sudden sensations of intense heat that typically start in the chest or face and then spread throughout the body. Hot flashes are thought to be triggered by changes in estrogen levels, which affect the body's thermostat, known as the hypothalamus. When estrogen levels drop, the hypothalamus perceives this as a signal that the body is overheating, leading to the dilation of blood vessels and increased blood flow to the skin, resulting in the sensation of heat and flushing. These episodes can occur unexpectedly, disrupting daily activities and causing discomfort and embarrassment for many women.

Mood swings are another common symptom of hormonal imbalance during menopause. Fluctuations in estrogen and progesterone levels can affect neurotransmitters in the brain, such as serotonin and dopamine, which play a crucial role in regulating mood. As hormone levels fluctuate, it can lead to disruptions in the delicate balance of these neurotransmitters, resulting in mood swings, irritability, anxiety, and even depression. Additionally, the psychological impact of experiencing symptoms like hot flashes and sleep disturbances can further exacerbate mood disturbances, creating a vicious cycle of emotional instability.

Sleep disturbances are also prevalent among menopausal women and are often linked to hormonal changes. Estrogen and progesterone play critical roles in regulating the sleep-wake cycle, and fluctuations in these hormones can disrupt the natural rhythm of sleep. For example, declining estrogen levels can lead to night sweats, which can awaken women from sleep and make it difficult to fall back asleep. Additionally, hormonal changes can contribute to other sleep disorders, such as insomnia and sleep apnea, further exacerbating sleep disturbances during menopause. The resulting sleep deprivation can have far-reaching consequences, affecting mood, cognitive function, and overall quality of life.

But here's where intermittent fasting enters the picture as a potential solution. Studies have shown that intermittent fasting can alleviate many of the symptoms associated with menopause, offering relief to women navigating this transformative phase.

One way intermittent fasting may alleviate menopausal symptoms is by promoting hormonal balance. A study published in the journal Cell Metabolism in 2017 found that intermittent fasting can improve insulin sensitivity and reduce insulin-like growth factor 1 (IGF-1) levels, which is associated with aging and age-related diseases. By improving insulin sensitivity and reducing IGF-1 levels, intermittent fasting may help regulate hormonal fluctuations contributing to symptoms like hot flashes and mood swings.

Additionally, intermittent fasting has been shown to reduce inflammation in the body, which may help alleviate symptoms such as joint pain and mood disturbances. A study published in Cell Research in 2020 demonstrated that intermittent fasting can activate cellular processes that enhance the body's ability to repair damaged DNA and reduce inflammation. By reducing inflammation, intermittent fasting may help alleviate symptoms associated with menopause, such as joint pain and mood swings.

Furthermore, intermittent fasting may support better sleep quality, indirectly alleviating menopausal symptoms like irritability and fatigue. A review published in the journal Nutrients in 2019 found that intermittent fasting can improve sleep quality by regulating circadian rhythms and promoting the production of melatonin, a hormone that regulates sleep-wake cycles. By improving sleep quality, intermittent fasting may help reduce symptoms like mood swings and irritability associated with sleep disturbances during menopause.

## Mood Enhancement and Emotional Well-being

Hormonal imbalances can impact emotional health beyond physical symptoms. Serotonin and dopamine are two key hormones involved in mood regulation, both of which play intricate roles in emotional well-being.

Hormones play a crucial role in regulating mood and emotional health, and their fluctuations can significantly impact women, particularly those over 50. Serotonin and dopamine, which play intricate roles in emotional well-being, are among the critical hormones in mood regulation.

Serotonin, often called the "feel-good" hormone, is a neurotransmitter that helps regulate mood, appetite, sleep, and other functions. Serotonin levels influence mood stability, feelings of happiness and well-being, and the ability to cope with stress. Dopamine, another neurotransmitter, is often associated with pleasure, reward, and motivation. It is critical in regulating mood, attention, learning, and movement. Its release is stimulated by rewarding experiences and reinforces behaviors associated with pleasure and satisfaction.

In women over 50, fluctuations in serotonin levels can occur due to various factors, including hormonal changes associated with menopause. Estrogen plays a role in serotonin synthesis and regulation. As estrogen levels decrease, serotonin levels may also fluctuate, leading to mood swings, irritability, anxiety, and even depression.

Like serotonin, dopamine levels can fluctuate in women over 50, contributing to mood and emotional well-being changes. Estrogen has been found to influence dopamine activity in the brain, and its decline during menopause can impact dopamine synthesis and signaling. This can lead to mood swings, decreased motivation, and a reduced sense of pleasure or reward.

Excitingly, intermittent fasting emerges as a promising avenue for enhancing mood and emotional well-being. In her article "Fasting and Depression: Benefits and Risks," Susan Fishman delves into a study involving fasting women who reported experiencing a profound sense of achievement, reward, pride, and control during fasting periods. Additionally, in the article "Role of therapeutic fasting in women's health: An overview" by Pradeep Nair and Pranav Khawale, fasting's impact on women's mental health, especially amid the challenges of menopause, is explored. The authors note that fasting has been linked to improved self-esteem, leading to a more positive mental outlook. Moreover, fasting has shown promise in reducing symptoms of anxiety and depression while enhancing social functioning. The therapeutic effects of fasting extend to diminishing stress levels and uplifting mood, as evidenced by increased vigilance and overall mood improvement reported by many clinicians (Fishman, n.d.; Nair & Khawale, n.d.).

## Practical Tips for Hormonal Balance Through Fasting

Now that we've explored the science behind intermittent fasting and hormonal health let's focus on practical implementation. If you're new to intermittent fasting or looking to optimize your fasting routine, here are a few tips to get you started:

- **Start slowly**: Ease into intermittent fasting by gradually extending your fasting window. Listen to your body and adjust your fasting schedule as needed.
- **Stay hydrated:** Drink plenty of water during fasting to stay hydrated and support cellular function.
- **Focus on nutrient-dense foods:** When breaking your fast, prioritize whole, nutrient-dense foods to nourish your body and support hormonal balance.
- **Seek support:** Join online communities or seek guidance from healthcare professionals to confidently navigate the intermittent fasting journey. Getting this book is a great start!
- **Choose the Right Method:** There are various intermittent fasting protocols, including the 16/8 method, the 5:2 method, or alternate-day fasting.

Experiment with different approaches to find the one that best suits your lifestyle and preferences. Chapter 5 will help you choose a method that is right for you.

- **Listen to Your Body:** Pay attention to how your body responds to fasting. Adjust your fasting schedule accordingly if you experience any adverse side effects or discomfort. It's essential to prioritize your health and well-being above all else.

As you embark on your intermittent fasting journey, remember that listening to your body and making adjustments as needed is essential. With patience, consistency, and a focus on overall health, intermittent fasting can be a powerful tool for achieving hormonal balance and improving your quality of life. In the next chapter, we'll delve into the importance of balanced recipes and meal plans to complement your intermittent fasting regimen. We'll provide practical tools and delicious recipes to help you nourish your body while supporting your hormonal health. Get ready to discover a new world of culinary delights that will enhance your fasting experience and energize and satisfy you.

THREE

# Balanced Recipes for Hormonal Health

---

" " *"Let food be thy medicine and medicine be thy food."*

Hippocrates

I n a world where fad diets come and go, it's easy to lose sight of the fundamental truth that Hippocrates eloquently expressed centuries ago. Food isn't just fuel; it's medicine for the body and soul. Embarking on the journey of intermittent fasting involves more than just abstaining from eating; it highlights the significance of intentional food choices. As mentioned before, the foods we consume during fasting windows play a pivotal role in determining the effectiveness of this approach, especially when we seek to maintain hormonal balance and overall well-being.

As we delve into this chapter, you can anticipate a curated collection of 50 recipes thoughtfully designed to align with the principles of intermittent fasting. Each recipe is crafted with the unique nutritional needs of women over 50, aiming for sustenance and a harmonious synergy with the fasting practice. These recipes are more than just meals; they are a holistic culinary toolkit, empowering you to make informed and health-conscious choices to support your journey toward hormonal balance and enhanced well-being. The ingredients in each recipe are designed to keep you healthy and satiated.

## Importance of Nutritional Balance

A balanced diet lays the foundation for optimal hormonal balance and overall health, especially for women over 50. A rich and varied diet, brimming with essential nutrients like vitamins, minerals, proteins, and healthy fats, becomes the conductor of this harmonious balance, ensuring our well-being from the inside out. Nutrient-rich foods provide the building blocks for hormone production, cellular repair, and metabolic function.

As women age, their nutritional needs change, and ensuring they are getting all the nutrients required for healthy aging becomes essential. However, many women in this age group may need more crucial nutrients due to dietary habits or age-related changes in metabolism. According to sources like AARP and Fortune, some essential nutrients that women over 50 may be deficient in include calcium, vitamin D, vitamin B12, vitamin B6, vitamin B9 (folate), vitamin E, and magnesium.

Calcium and vitamin D are essential for bone health and reducing the risk of osteoporosis. Vitamin B12, B6, and folate are vital for maintaining cognitive function, energy levels, and heart health. Vitamin E is an antioxidant that helps protect cells from damage caused by free radicals. At the same time, magnesium plays a role in muscle and nerve function, blood sugar regulation, and bone health.

We help fill these nutrient gaps through the food we consume by incorporating ingredients rich in these essential nutrients. For example, milk, yogurt, and cheese are excellent sources of calcium and vitamin D. Leafy green vegetables, legumes, and fortified cereals can provide folate. At the same time, lean meats, fish, and poultry are good vitamin B12 and B6 sources. Additionally, Nuts, seeds, and vegetable oils are rich in vitamin E, as well as whole grains, nuts, seeds, and leafy green vegetables, which are excellent sources of magnesium.

Our collection of recipes is carefully crafted to address these nutritional gaps and promote hormonal equilibrium. From antioxidant-rich fruits and vegetables to lean proteins and healthy fats, each recipe is thoughtfully designed to provide a comprehensive array of essential nutrients. By incorporating these recipes into your meal plan, you can ensure your body receives the nourishment needed to thrive.

Beyond specific nutrients, embracing variety is the key to a resilient and well-supported body. Make your plate a canvas of colors, incorporating a spectrum of fruits, vegetables, and protein sources. This diverse palette enhances nutritional intake and introduces myriad flavors to daily meals.

## Meal Timing and Scheduling

Meal timing is crucial in optimizing the benefits of intermittent fasting, particularly for women over 50. Understanding how to structure your meals around your fasting schedule is vital to maximizing the effectiveness of this approach.

One can consider several fasting schedules, depending on one's preferences and lifestyle. One popular method is the 16/8 protocol, which involves fasting for 16 hours and eating within an 8-hour window daily. This schedule allows for flexibility in meal timing while still providing the benefits of intermittent fasting. Another option is the 5:2 method, which involves eating normally five days a week and restricting calorie intake to 500-600 calories on two non-consecutive days. This approach may suit women who prefer a less restrictive fasting schedule.

When it comes to adjusting meal timing based on fasting schedules, lifestyle factors, and hormonal needs, there are several strategies women over 50 can employ. For example, some women may find it helpful to schedule their fasting periods when they are less active or busy, such as in the morning or early afternoon. This can help minimize hunger and discomfort during fasting hours. Additionally, women can experiment with different meal timing strategies to see what works best for them. For example, some prefer larger meals during their eating window, while others prefer smaller, more frequent meals. It's essential to listen to your body and adjust your meal timing accordingly.

It's also important to consider how meal timing can impact hormone levels. For example, eating carbohydrate-rich meals during the eating window can lead to fluctuations in insulin levels, which may affect blood sugar regulation and energy levels. Women can support stable hormone levels and overall health by focusing on nutrient-dense foods and balanced meals.

In chapter five, we'll explore different fasting schedules in more depth and offer practical tips on how to align your meal timing with your fasting goals. Whether you're an early riser who prefers breakfast or a night owl who enjoys late-night snacks, we'll help you find a meal schedule that works for you. By mastering the art of meal timing, you can enhance the efficacy of intermittent fasting and unlock its full potential for hormonal balance.

## 50 Healthy, Balanced Recipes

Now, let's dive into the heart of this chapter: our collection of 50 healthy and balanced recipes designed to nourish your body and soul. From hearty breakfasts to satisfying dinners and everything in between, these recipes offer diverse flavors and textures to tantalize your taste buds and keep you satisfied throughout your fasting journey.

Each recipe is crafted with hormonal health in mind, incorporating nutrient-dense ingredients that support hormonal balance and overall well-being. Whether you're craving a comforting bowl of soup, a salad bursting with fresh produce, or a decadent dessert to satisfy your sweet tooth, we've got you covered. With options to suit every palate and dietary preference, you'll never have to sacrifice flavor for health again.

As we embark on this culinary adventure, remember that food is more than just sustenance; it's a source of nourishment, joy, and connection. So, let's savor each bite, celebrate nature's abundance of flavors, and nourish our bodies with the love and care they deserve.

## *10 Reasons to Break Your Fast*

### Poached Egg on Avacado Toast

Perfectly poached eggs, a top creamy avocado mash, for a delightful breakfast indulgence.

**Time:** 15 minutes
**Serving Size:** 1 slice
**Servings Per Recipe**: 4
**Prep Time:** 10 minutes
**Cook Time:** 5 minutes
**Nutritional Facts:**

| Calories | 440kcal |
|----------|---------|
| Carbs    | 27g     |
| Fat      | 31g     |
| Protein  | 16g     |

**Ingredients:**

- 4 eggs
- 2 ripe avocados
- 2 teaspoons lemon juice (or juice of 1 lime)
- 4 slices thick bread
- 1 cup cheese (grated, edam, gruyere or whatever you have on hand)
- salt & freshly ground black pepper
- 4 teaspoons butter (for spreading on toast)

**Directions:**

1. Poach eggs using your favourite method.
2. Meanwhile, cut the avocados in half and remove the pit.
3. Using a spoon scoop out the flesh into a bowl
4. Season avocado with lemon or lime juice and salt & pepper.
5. Mash roughly using a fork.
6. Toast the bread and spread with butter.
7. Spread the avocado mix onto each slice of buttered toast and top each with a poached egg.
8. Sprinkle over the grated cheese and serve immediately.

## Breakfast Frittata

The only thing better than ham and eggs for breakfast: baked ham and eggs.

**Time:** 45 minutes
**Serving Size:** 8oz
**Servings Per Recipe:** 6
**Prep Time:** 10 minutes
**Cook Time:** 25 minutes
**Nutritional Facts:**

| Calories | 260kcal |
|----------|---------|
| Carbs | 14g |
| Fat | 15g |
| Protein | 18g |

**Ingredients:**

- 2 cups potatoes (cut into small cubes)
- 1 cup cooked ham (cut into small cubes)
- ½ cup onion (finely chopped)
- 8 eggs
- 4 egg whites
- 2 tsp baking powder
- 1 green onion (sliced)
- 1 cup low-fat cheddar cheese (grated)
- 2 tbsp olive oil

## Directions:

1. Saute potato, onion, and ham in olive oil in an oven-safe pan until the potato becomes soft.
2. In a separate bowl hisk egg whites, eggs, and baking powder until frothy.
3. Add green onion to the pan.
4. Pour egg mixture into pan and top with cheese.
5. Place the pan in the oven and bake for 35 minutes or until eggs are set.
6. Season with salt and pepper and serve hot or cold.

### Broccoli Quiche

A delightful blend of beaten eggs, fresh vegetables, and cheese baked to perfection creating a hearty and satisfying breakfast.

**Time:** 55 minutes
**Serving Size:** 10oz
**Serving Per Recipe:**6
**Prep Time:** 5 minutes
**Cook Time:** 50 minutes
**Nutritional Facts:**

| Calories | 190kcal |
|----------|---------|
| Carbs | 20g |
| Fat | 7g |
| Protein | 11g |

**Ingredients:**

- 1 cup egg (beaten)
- 1 ½ cups low-fat milk
- ¾ cup Bisquick low-fat baking mix
- 1 tsp salt
- ¼ tsp ground black pepper
- 2 garlic cloves (minced)
- 2 ½ cups broccoli/spinach (finely chopped)
- 1 medium onion (finely chopped)
- 1 medium red pepper (finely chopped)
- ½ cups low-fat mozzarella cheese
- Cooking spray

**Directions:**

1. Preheat the oven to 400 °F.
2. Blend eggs, milk, Bisquick, salt and pepper, and garlic until smooth.
3. In an oven-safe pan, saute half of the broccoli until partly brown.
4. Once partly brown, add the remaining broccoli, half onion, red pepper, and cheese to the pan and simmer for 5 minutes.
5. Remove from heat and pour the egg mixture on top, followed by the rest of the ingredients except the cheese.
6. Place the (now filled) oven-safe pan in the oven and bake for 45 minutes or until eggs are set and lightly browned.
7. Add the cheese and bake for another 5 minutes

8. Wait until cool before dividing into 6 slices and enjoy with optional sour cream as a topping.

## Protein Pancakes

Nutritious and protein-packed pancakes for a healthy breakfast option.

**Time:** 20minutes
**Serving Size:** 3 pancakes
**Serving Per Recipe:**3
**Prep Time:** 10 minutes
**Cook Time:** 10 minutes
**Nutritional Facts:**

| Calories | 258kcal |
|----------|---------|
| Carbs | 37g |
| Fat | 3g |
| Protein | 14g |

**Ingredients:**

- 1 cup oats
- 1 banana
- 2 eggs
- ½ cup egg whites
- 1 teaspoon baking powder
- a pinch of salt

- a pinch of cinnamon
- 2 scoops protein powder *(29 grams)*
- 2 tablespoons flax meal

**Directions:**

1. Combine all the ingredients in a blender and blend until smooth
2. Heat a pan on medium high heat. Spray with non stick spray
3. Add batter in small circles – about 1/4 cup per pancake.
4. Sprinkle with blueberries or chocolate chips (optional) When the edges start to look brown (2-3 minutes), flip and cook for another minute or two on the other side.
5. Add any additional toppings of your choice.

### Cabbage Scramble

This recipe marries the quick-cooking prowess of eggs and cabbage with the rich flavor of sautéed onions.

**Time:** 15 minutes
**Serving Size:** 1(182g)
**Serving Per Recipe:** 2
**Prep Time:** 5 minutes
**Cook Time:** 10 minutes

**Nutritional Facts:**

| Calories | 300kcal |
|----------|---------|
| Carbs | 10g |
| Fat | 25g |
| Protein | 15g |

**Ingredients:**

- 2-3 scrambled eggs
- ½ tbsp grass-fed butter
- 1-2 cup chopped cabbage
- ¼ - ½ cup sliced onions
- Pinch of sea salt
- 1 tsp pumpkin seeds
- 1oz sharp cheddar (optional)

**Directions:**

1. Toss half of the butter, sliced onions, chopped cabbage, a pinch of sea salt, and pepper in a non-stick pan. Cook for a few minutes.
2. In the same pan, add the remaining butter and two eggs. Scramble and cook until they reach your desired level of doneness.
3. Then, slide your scrambled eggs into your cabbage group before mixing thoroughly.

4. Top the mixture with pumpkin seeds and, if desired, a sprinkle of sharp cheddar for an extra shot of flavor and nutrition.

### Greek Yogurt and Berry Bowl

A bowl of Greek yogurt adorned with a mix of fresh berries provides a simple yet delightful morning treat rich in protein and antioxidants.

**Time:** 5–7 minutes
**Serving Size:** 1 bowl
**Prep Time:** 5–7 minutes
**Cook Time:** No cooking required
**Nutritional Facts:**

| Calories | 200kcal |
|----------|---------|
| Carb | 20g |
| Fats | 9g |
| Protein | 12g |

**Ingredients:**

- 1 cup unsweetened Greek yogurt
- ½ cup mixed berries (blueberries, strawberries, raspberries)
- 1 tbsp honey (optional for sweetness)
- ½ oz chopped nuts (almonds, walnuts, or your choice)

- ⅓ oz chia seeds (optional for added crunch and nutrition)

**Directions:**

1. Spoon the Greek yogurt into a bowl.

2. Rinse the mixed berries and place them over the yogurt.

3. Drizzle honey over the yogurt and berries if you prefer a touch of sweetness.

4. Sprinkle chopped nuts and chia seeds for extra texture and nutritional goodness.

### Shakshuka with Greens

Indulge in a flavorful medley of spiced chickpeas, hearty greens, and perfectly cooked eggs in this satisfying skillet meal.

**Time:** 25 minutes
**Serving Size:** 1 egg
**Servings Per Recipe**: 4
**Prep Time:** 10 minutes
**Cook Time:** 35 minutes

**Nutritional Facts:**

| Calories | 380kcal |
|----------|---------|
| Carbs | 25g |
| Fat | 22g |
| Protein | 20g |

**Ingredients:**

- 4 tbsp olive oil, divided
- 1 medium red onion, cut into ½ -inch pieces
- 1 medium red bell pepper, cut into ½ -inch pieces
- 2 cups sliced white button mushrooms
- 2 tsp Garlic Powder
- 1 ½ tsp Ground Cumin
- 1 ½ tsp Ground Coriander
- ½ tsp Smoked Paprika
- ½ tsp salt
- ¼ tsp Crushed Red Pepper
- 1 ½ cups finely chopped plum tomatoes
- 1 can (15 ounces) chickpeas, drained and rinsed
- 3 cups kale, stems removed and cut into 1-inch pieces
- 3 cups baby spinach, packed
- ½ cup unsalted vegetable stock
- 4 eggs
- ¼ cup crumbled feta cheese

**Directions:**

1. Preheat the oven to 375°F (190°F).
2. Heat 2 tablespoons of the oil in a large skillet on medium heat.
3. Add mushrooms, onion and pepper; cook and stir for 5 minutes or until softened.
4. Add remaining 2 tablespoons oil, spices, salt and red pepper.
5. Stir in tomatoes and chickpeas.
6. Add kale and spinach, in batches, cooking until wilted before each addition.
7. Add in stock; cook for a couple minutes.
8. Divide mixture among 4 small dishes/skillets.Use the back of a large spoon to create a well in the center of each portion. Crack one egg into each well.
9. Bake 8 to 10 minutes or until eggs are desired doneness.
10. Sprinkle feta cheese on top

**Blueberry Pecan Overnight Oats**

Start your day with a delightful blend of creamy oats, sweet blueberries, and crunchy pecans in this easy-to-make overnight breakfast.

**Time:** 8 hours and 10 minutes
**Serving Size:** 1 jar/bowl
**Prep Time:** 8 hours (overnight)
**Cook Time:** 10 minutes

## Nutritional Facts:

| Calories | 291kcal |
|----------|---------|
| Carbs | 49g |
| Fat | 8g |
| Protein | 9g |

## Ingredients:

- 1 ½ cup old-fashioned rolled oats
- ½ cup water
- Pinch of salt
- ½ cup blueberries, fresh or frozen
- 2 tablespoons nonfat plain Greek yogurt
- 1 tbsp toasted chopped pecans
- 2 tsp pure maple syrup

## Directions:

1. Add oats, water and salt in a jar or bowl.
2. Cover and refrigerate overnight.
3. In the morning, heat if desired, and top with blueberries, yogurt, pecans and syrup.

## Tropical Acai Bowl

Indulge in the refreshing flavors of the tropics with this vibrant smoothie bowl, featuring acai berry puree, sweet banana, tangy pineapple, and creamy coconut milk.

**Time:** 5 minutes
**Serving Size:** 8.5oz
**Serving Per Recipe:** 2
**Prep Time:** 5 minutes
**Cook Time:** No cooking required!
**Nutritional Facts:**

| Calories | 222kcal |
|----------|---------|
| Carbs | 22g |
| Fat | 14g |
| Protein | 2g |

**Ingredients:**

- 7oz frozen unsweetened pure acai berry puree
- ½ cup frozen banana slices
- ½ cup frozen pineapple chunks
- ½ cup Unsweetened Coconut Milk
- 1 tbsp Vanilla Extract

**Directions:**

1. Combine acai puree, banana, pineapple, coconut milk and vanilla in a blender.
2. Blend until smooth.
3. Transfer mixture to serving bowls
4. Top with any fruit and garnishes, as desired.

### Chocolate Quinoa Bowl

Indulge in a velvety chocolate-quinoa delight, blending quinoa flakes, cocoa powder, almond milk, and vanilla protein powder, topped with creamy coconut yogurt and decadent dark chocolate chips for a guilt-free treat.

**Time:** 5 minutes
**Serving Size:** 1 bowl
**Prep Time:** 2 minutes
**Cook Time:** 3 minutes
**Nutritional Facts:**

| Calories | 482kcal |
|----------|---------|
| Carbs | 73g |
| Fat | 15g |
| Protein | 19g |

**Ingredients:**

- 1/4 cup quinoa flakes
- 2 tablespoons unsweetened cocoa powder
- 1/2 cup unsweetened almond milk
- 1/2 scoop vanilla protein powder
- 1/2 cup water
- 1 medium banana mashed
- 2 tablespoons coconut yogurt (for topping)
- 2 tablespoons dark chocolate chips (for topping)

**Directions:**

1. Combine all ingredients into a small saucepan.
2. Whisk until mixed well.
3. Bring mixture to a boil, then reduce to a high simmer for 2-3minutes.
4. Transfer to a bowl, top with yogurt and chocolate chips, and enjoy!

*10 Nourishing Lunch Options*

### Lemon and Herb-Crusted Salmon

Salmon fillets delicately coated in a medley of fragrant herbs.

**Time:** 1 hour and 20 minutes
**Serving Size:** 1 fillet
**Servings Per Recipe**: 4
**Prep Time:** 1 hour
**Cook Time:** 20 minutes

**Nutritional Facts:**

| Calories | 381kcal |
|----------|---------|
| Carbs | 17g |
| Fat | 18g |
| Protein | 37g |

**Ingredients:**

- 2 tsp fresh dill
- ½ tsp pepper
- ½ tsp salt
- ½ tsp garlic powder
- 1 ½ lbs salmon (about 4 fillets)
- ½ cup packed brown sugar
- 1 chicken bouillon cube, mixed with
- 3 tbsp water
- 3 tbsp oil
- 3 tbsp soy sauce
- 4 tbsp finely chopped green onions
- 1 lemon, thinly sliced
- 2 slices onions, seperated into rings

**Directions:**

1. Sprinkle dill, pepper, salt and garlic powder over salmon.
2. Place in a shallow glass pan.

3. Mix sugar, chicken boullion, oil, soy sauce, and green onions.
4. Pour over salmon.
5. Cover and chill for 1 hour, turn once halfway.
6. Drain and discard marinade.
7. Put on a grill on medium heat, place a slice of lemon and onion on top.
8. Cover and cook for 15 minutes, or until the fish is done.

### Cheesy Chicken Salad

Wholesome chicken salad with crisp veggies, creamy dressing, and cheddar.

**Time:** 40 minutes
**Serving Size:** 1 bowl
**Prep Time:** 45 minutes
**Cook Time:** No cooking required!
**Nutritional Facts:**

| Calories | 364kcal |
|----------|---------|
| Carbs | 15g |
| Fat | 9g |
| Protein | 53.2g |

**Ingredients:**

- 1 cup cooked boneless skinless chicken breast, cubed
- ¼ cup celery, finely chopped
- ¼ cup carrot, shredded
- ½ cup Baby Spinach, roughly chopped
- 2 ½ Tbsp light mayonnaise
- 2 Tbsp nonfat sour cream
- ⅛ tsp dried parsley
- 2 tsp Dijon mustard
- ¼ cup reduced-fat sharp cheddar cheese, shredded

**Directions:**

1. Combine all ingredients in a bowl
2. Mix well so everything is coated.
3. Chill in the fridge for at least 30 minutes

### Citrus Mahi Mahi Crunch

Succulent mahi-mahi fillets kissed with lemon, seasoned with garlic and pepper, coated in a creamy onion-infused mayonnaise, and delicately crusted with breadcrumbs for a tantalizing crunch.

**Time:** 30 minutes
**Serving Size:** 1 fillet
**Servings Per Recipe**: 4
**Prep Time:** 5 minutes
**Cook Time:** 25 minutes

## Nutritional Facts:

| Calories | 201kcal |
|----------|---------|
| Carbs | 3g |
| Fat | 14g |
| Protein | 42g |

## Ingredients:

- 4 fillets Mahi Mahi fish (2lbs)
- 1 lemon, juiced
- 1/4 tsp garlic salt
- 1/4 tsp ground black pepper
- 1 cup mayonnaise
- 1/4 cup white onion, finely chopped
- 1/4 cup breadcrumbs

## Directions:

1. Preheat the oven to 425°F.
2. Rinse fish and put in a baking dish.
3. Squeeze lemon juice on fish then sprinkle with garlic salt and pepper.
4. Mix mayonnaise and chopped onions and spread on fish.
5. Sprinkle with breadcrumbs and bake for 25 minutes.

## Baked Potato

Achieving the ideal combination of a crispy skin and irresistibly soft flesh, This classic baked potato is a versatile canvas ready to be adorned with your favorite toppings.

**Time:** 1 hour 10 minutes
**Serving Size:** 1
**Prep Time:** 10 minutes
**Cook Time:** 1 hour
**Nutritional Facts:**

| Calories | 369kcal |
|----------|---------|
| Carbs | 65g |
| Fat | .5gs |
| Protein | 8g |

**Ingredients:**

- 1 large russet potato
- 1/4 cup canola oil
- pinch of kosher salt

**Directions:**

1. Preheat the oven to 350 °F and position racks in the top and bottom thirds.
2. Wash the russet potato thoroughly with cold running water.
3. Dry the potato well and use a fork to poke 8–12 deep holes all over
4. Lightly coat the potato with canola oil.
5. Sprinkle kosher salt over the potato and place it directly on the rack in the middle of the oven.
6. Put a baking sheet (or a piece of aluminum foil) on the lower rack to catch any drippings.
7. Bake for 1 hour or until the skin feels crisp but the flesh beneath feels soft.
8. Cut open and add your desired toppings.

## Sauerkraut Salad

Zesty sauerkraut salad with crunchy veggies, sweet-tangy dressing perfection.

**Time:** 8 hours and 15 minutes
**Serving Size:** 1 (146 g)
**Servings Per Recipe**: 6
**Prep Time:** 15 minutes
**Cook/Chill Time:** 8 hours in fridge(overnight)

**Nutritional Facts:**

| Calories | 224kcal |
|----------|---------|
| Carbs | 30g |
| Fat | 12g |
| Protein | 1g |

**Ingredients:**

- 1 can sauerkraut (drained)
- 1 cup celery (finely chopped)
- 1/2 cup green pepper (finely chopped)
- 2 tbsp onions (finely chopped)
- 1/2 tsp salt
- 1/2 tsp pepper
- 3/4 cup sugar
- 1/3 cup salad oil
- 1/3 cup cider or 1/3 cup white vinegar

**Directions:**

1. In a large bowl, mix the vegetables and sauerkraut.
2. Heat the oil, sugar, salt, pepper, and cider/vinegar until sugar dissolves.
3. Allow to cool slightly and pour over vegetables and sauerkraut.
4. Chill in the fridge overnight, tossing before plating, and serve cold.

## Greek Salad Wrap

Mediterranean wrap bursting with chickpeas, veggies, and tangy vinaigrette.

**Time:** 15 minutes
**Serving Size:** 1 wrap
**Servings Per Recipe**: 4
**Prep Time:** 15 minutes
**Cook Time:** No cooking required!
**Nutritional Facts:**

| Calories | 460kcal |
|----------|---------|
| Carbs | 50g |
| Fat | 23g |
| Protein | 14g |

**Ingredients:**

- 2 ½ tbsp. red wine vinegar
- ¼ cup olive oil
- Kosher salt and pepper
- 1 15-oz can chickpeas, rinsed
- 2 cup cherry tomatoes, halved

- 1 small English cucumber, cubed
- ¼ cup Kalamata olives, roughly chopped
- ¼ small red onion, thinly sliced
- ¼ cup crumbled feta cheese
- 2 cups baby spinach
- 4 10-inch wraps

**Directions:**

1. In a medium bowl, whisk together vinegar, oil, and 1/2 teaspoon each salt and pepper.
2. Add chickpeas, tomatoes, cucumber, olives, red onion and toss.
3. Add feta crumbles
4. Evenly divide baby spinach among wraps
5. Top with chickpea salad and roll tightly.

**Black Bean Soup**

Savory black bean soup with cumin, garlic, and vibrant garnishes.

**Time:** 25 minutes
**Serving Size:** 1(329g)
**Servings Per Recipe**: 4
**Prep Time:** 5 minutes
**Cook Time:** 20 minutes

**Nutritional Facts:**

| Calories | 331kcal |
|----------|---------|
| Carbs | 41g |
| Fat | 12g |
| Protein | 17g |

**Ingredients:**

- 3 tbsp olive oil
- 1 medium onion (chopped)
- 1 tbsp ground cumin
- 2–3 cloves garlic
- 2 cans black beans
- 2 cups vegetable broth
- salt and pepper
- 1 small red onion (finely chopped)
- ¼ cup cilantro (coarsely chopped)

**Directions:**

1. In a medium pan, saute the onions until translucent.
2. Add cumin and stir 30 seconds,
3. Add the garlic and cook for 1 minute
4. Add 1 can of the beans and the vegetable broth.
5. Allow to simmer, stirring often
6. Remove from heat.
7. Blend the mixture until smooth

8. Return to the pot and add the second can of beans. Stir well and heat if cold.
9. Top with red onion and cilantro to garnish

**Veggie Delight Sandwich**

Vibrant veggie toast with creamy avocado, hummus, and wholesome toppings.

**Time:** 30 minutes
**Serving Size:** 1 Sandwich
**Servings Per Recipe**: 4
**Prep Time:** 20 minutes
**Cook Time:** 10 minutes
**Nutritional Facts:**

| Calories | 504kcal |
|----------|---------|
| Carbs | 53g |
| Fat | 28g |
| Protein | 17g |

**Ingredients:**

- 1 small eggplant, sliced 1/2 inch thick, or 8 portobello mushroom
- 1 ½ tbsp. olive oil if using eggplant (or 3 tbsp. if using portobellos)
- Kosher salt and pepper

- 2 ripe avocados
- 2 tbsp. fresh lemon juice
- ¼ tsp. red pepper flakes
- 8 slices whole-grain bread, lightly toasted
- 1 cup hummus, divided
- 2 cup baby arugula, divided
- Pinch of Flaky salt
- 1 large heirloom tomato, sliced 1/4 inch thick, divided
- ½ large English cucumber, chopped
- 2 cups sprouts of choice (such as broccoli, radish, or sunflower), divided

**Directions:**

1. Heat broiler to 450°F
2. On a rimmed baking sheet, brush both sides of eggplant or mushrooms with oil
3. Season with 1/4 teaspoon salt and pepper.
4. Broil 4 to 7 minutes until tender and browned in spots,
5. Meanwhile, in a medium bowl, mash avocados with lemon juice, red pepper flakes, and 1/2 teaspoon each salt and pepper.
6. Spread 4 slices of toast with mashed avocados and remaining 4 slices with hummus
7. Add fillings on top to make sandwiches, sprinkling flaky salt on tomato.

## Shrimp and Soba Noodle Salad

Delicate soba noodles intertwined with vibrant veggies and succulent shrimp, topped with zesty ginger dressing.

**Time:** 20 minutes
**Serving Size:** 1 bowl
**Prep Time:** 5 minutes
**Cook Time:** 15 minutes
**Nutritional Facts:**

| Calories | 555kcal |
|----------|---------|
| Carbs | 62g |
| Fat | 18g |
| Protein | 42g |

**Ingredients:**

- 2 oz. soba noodles
- ¼ cup frozen shelled edamame
- 2 oz. purple cabbage thinly sliced
- 1 small carrot, peeled and cut into 1/2-inch pieces
- ½ tbsp. finely grated fresh ginger
- 1 tbsp. rice vinegar
- ¼ tbsp. reduced-sodium soy sauce
- ½ tsp. light brown sugar
- 1 tbsp. canola oil
- 4 oz. cooked large peeled and deveined shrimp

- 1 scallions, thinly sliced

**Directions:**

1. Cook noodles per package directions,
2. Adding edamame during the last minute of cooking.
3. Drain, run under cold water to cool, then transfer back to the pot.
4. Meanwhile, in a food processor add carrot, ginger, vinegar, soy sauce, and sugar and pulse until finely chopped. With the processor running, slowly add oil until fully incorporated. Divide between two tiny containers.
5. Combine noodles and edamame, cabbage, shrimp and scallions in a bowl.
6. Add the dressing on top.

*10 Dinners to Dine For*

**Rosemary Walnut Crusted Salmon**

Nutrient-rich salmon with a flavorful crust, a simple and satisfying choice.

**Time:** 20 minutes
**Serving Size:** 3oz
**Servings Per Recipe**: 4
**Prep Time:** 10 minutes
**Cook Time:** 10 minutes

**Nutritional Facts:**

| Calories | 222kcal |
|----------|---------|
| Carbs | 4g |
| Fat | 12g |
| Protein | 24g |

**Ingredients:**

- 2 tsp Dijon mustard
- 1 clove garlic, minced
- ¼ tsp lemon zest
- 1 tsp lemon juice
- 1 tsp chopped fresh rosemary
- ½ tsp honey
- ½ tsp kosher salt
- ¼ tsp crushed red pepper
- 3 tbsp panko breadcrumbs
- 3 tbsp finely chopped walnuts
- 1 tsp extra-virgin olive oil
- 1 lbs salmon fillet
- Cooking spray
- fresh parsley and lemon wedges (garnish)

**Directions:**

1. Preheat the oven to 425°F. Line a large rimmed baking sheet with parchment paper.
2. Mix mustard, garlic, lemon zest, lemon juice, rosemary, honey, salt and crushed red pepper in a small bowl.
3. Combine panko, walnuts and oil in another small bowl.
4. Place salmon on the prepared baking sheet. Spread the mustard mixture over the fish
5. Then sprinkle with the panko mixture, pressing to adhere.
6. Lightly coat with cooking spray.
7. Bake until the fish flakes easily with a fork ( 8 to 12 minutes) depending on thickness.
8. Sprinkle with parsley and serve with lemon wedges (Optional)

### Cheesy Spinach Cod Delight

Simple yet flavorful cod with spinach, tomato, mozzarella, seasoned to perfection.

**Time:** 20 minutes
**Serving Size:** 1 fillet
**Prep Time:** 10 minutes
**Cook Time:** 10 minutes

**Nutritional Facts:**

| Calories | 308kcal |
|----------|---------|
| Carbs | 6g |
| Fat | 19g |
| Protein | 28g |

**Ingredients:**

- 1 (4 oz) fillet cod
- salt and ground black pepper to taste
- 1 pinch garlic powder, or to taste
- ¼ cup roughly chopped spinach, or to taste
- ¼ tomato, diced
- 1 tbsp chopped onion
- 1 tbsp olive oil, or to taste
- 1 tbsp balsamic vinegar, or to taste
- 1 slice mozzarella cheese, cut into cubes

**Directions:**

1. Preheat an outdoor grill for medium-high heat.
2. Place cod on a piece of aluminum foil and season with salt, black pepper, and garlic powder.
3. Top cod with spinach, tomato, and onion; season again with salt and black pepper.
4. Drizzle olive oil and balsamic vinegar over cod and top with mozzarella cheese.

5. Fold foil over cod creating a packet, crimping the edges together making a seal.
6. Cook on the preheated grill until the fish flakes easily with a fork, 7 to 9 minutes.

### Filipino Ginger Garlic Chicken Soup (Tinola)

Invigorating soup melding ginger, chicken, papaya, and vibrant greens.

**Time:** 40 minutes
**Serving Size:** 1½ cups
**Servings Per Recipe**: 4
**Prep Time:** 20 minutes
**Cook Time:** 20 minutes
**Nutritional Facts:**

| Calories | 344kcal |
|----------|---------|
| Carbs | 21g |
| Fat | 14g |
| Protein | 27g |

**Ingredients:**

- 3 tbsp avocado oil
- ½ cup chopped yellow onion
- ¼ cup thinly sliced fresh ginger
- 6 cloves garlic, minced

- 1 lbs boneless, skinless chicken thighs, cut into 1/2-inch pieces
- 4 cups low-sodium chicken broth
- 1 ½ cups peeled and cubed green papaya
- 2 cups chopped bok choy leaves
- 1 tbsp fish sauce
- ¼ tsp salt
- ¼ tsp ground black pepper

**Directions:**

1. Heat oil in a large pot over medium heat.
2. Add onion, ginger and garlic; cook, stirring, until the onion starts to turn translucent,( 3 minutes).
3. Add chicken and broth; cook, stirring, until the chicken is just cooked through(5 minutes).
4. Add papaya and bok choy, fish sauce, salt and pepper; continue simmering until the vegetables are tender and the flavors have melded(5 minutes more).

### Stuffed Pepper Philly Cheesesteak

A classic Philly cheesesteak stuffed in a colorful bell pepper

**Time:** 1 hour
**Serving Size:** ½ stuffed pepper
**Servings Per Recipe**: 4
**Prep Time:** 10 minutes
**Cook Time:** 50 minutes

**Nutritional Facts:**

| Calories | 308kcal |
|----------|---------|
| Carbs | 12g |
| Fat | 17g |
| Protein | 29g |

**Ingredients:**

- 2 large bell peppers, halved
- 1 tbsp extra-virgin olive oil
- 1 large onion, sliced
- 8oz mushrooms, thinly sliced
- 12 oz top round steak, thinly sliced
- 1 tbsp Italian seasoning
- ½ tsp ground pepper
- ¼ tsp salt
- 1 tbsp Worcestershire sauce
- 4 slices provolone cheese

**Directions:**

1. Preheat the oven to 375°F.
2. Place pepper halves on a rimmed baking sheet. Bake until tender but still holding their shape, about 30 minutes.
3. Meanwhile, heat oil in a large skillet over medium heat.

4. Add onion and cook, stirring, until starting to brown(4 to 5 minutes).
5. Add mushrooms and cook, stirring, until they're softened and release their juices (about 5 minutes more).
6. Add steak, Italian seasoning, pepper and salt; cook, stirring, until the steak is just cooked through(3 to 5 minutes more).
7. Remove from heat and stir in Worcestershire.
8. Preheat the broiler too high. Divide the filling between the pepper halves and top each with a slice of cheese.
9. Broil 5 inches from the heat until the cheese is melted and lightly browned (2 to 3 minutes).

### Sheet Pan Chicken Fajitas

Simple sheet-pan chicken fajitas: easy prep, bold flavors, minimal cleanup.

**Time:** 40 minutes.
**Serving Size:** 2 fajitas
**Servings Per Recipe**: 4
**Prep Time:** 20 minutes
**Cook Time:** 20 minutes

**Nutritional Facts:**

| Calories | 357kcal |
|----------|---------|
| Carbs | 33g |
| Fat | 12g |
| Protein | 30g |

**Ingredients:**

- 1 lbs boneless, skinless chicken breasts
- 2 tbsp extra-virgin olive oil
- 1 tbsp chili powder
- 2 tsp ground cumin
- 1 tsp garlic powder
- ¾ tsp salt
- 1 large red bell pepper, sliced
- 1 large yellow bell pepper, sliced
- 1 large onion (red or white), sliced
- 1 tbsp lime juice
- 8 corn tortillas, warmed
- Lime wedges, cilantro, sour cream, avocado and/or pico de gallo for serving(optional)

**Directions:**

1. Preheat the oven to 400°F. Coat a large rimmed baking sheet with cooking spray.

2. Cut chicken breasts in half horizontally, then slice into strips.
3. Mix oil, chili powder, cumin, garlic powder and salt in a large bowl. Add the chicken and stir to coat with the spice mixture.
4. Add bell peppers and onion and stir to combine. Transfer the chicken and vegetables to the prepared baking sheet and spread in an even layer.
5. Roast on the middle rack for 15 minutes.
6. Leave the pan there and turn the broiler to high. Broil until the chicken is cooked through and the vegetables are browning in spots, about 5 minutes more.
7. Remove from the oven. Squeeze lime juice on top..
8. Serve the chicken and vegetables in warmed tortillas topping of choice (ex. cilantro, sour cream, avocado and/or pico de gallo)

### Lemon Garlic Chicken Pasta

Tender chicken, spinach, and lemon pasta with Parmesan perfection.

**Time:** 25 minutes
**Serving Size:** 2 cups
**Servings Per Recipe**: 4
**Prep Time:** 5 minutes
**Cook Time:** 20 minutes

**Nutritional Facts:**

| Calories | 335kcal |
|----------|---------|
| Carbs | 25g |
| Fat | 12g |
| Protein | 29g |

**Ingredients:**

- 8 oz penne pasta or whole-wheat penne pasta
- 2 tbsp extra-virgin olive oil
- 1 lbs boneless, skinless chicken breast or thighs,
- ½ teaspoon salt
- ¼ tsp ground pepper
- 4 cloves garlic, minced
- ½ cup dry white wine
- Juice and zest of 1 lemon
- 10 cups chopped fresh spinach
- 4 tbsp grated Parmesan cheese, divided

**Directions:**

1. Cook pasta according to package directions. Drain and set aside.
2. Meanwhile, heat oil in a large high-sided skillet over medium-high heat.
3. Add chicken, salt and pepper; cook, stirring occasionally, until just cooked through, 5 to 7

minutes.

4. Add garlic and cook, stirring, until fragrant, about 1
   minute. Stir in wine, lemon juice and zest; bring to a
   simmer.
5. Remove from heat. Stir in spinach and the cooked
   pasta. Cover and let stand until the spinach is just
   wilted.
6. Top each serving with 1 tbsp Parmesan.

**Beef & Mushroom Pasta Skillet**

Hearty beef and mushroom skillet pasta, nutritious and
comforting meal.

**Time:** 50 minutes
**Serving Size:** 1¼ cups
**Servings Per Recipe**: 4
**Prep Time:** 10 minutes
**Cook Time:** 40 minutes
**Nutritional Facts:**

| Calories | 582kcal |
|----------|---------|
| Carbs | 55g |
| Fat | 21g |
| Protein | 44g |

**Ingredients:**

- 1 tbsp extra-virgin olive oil
- 1 lbs 90% lean ground beef
- 8 oz mushrooms, finely chopped
- ½ cup diced onion
- 1 15-oz can added tomato sauce
- 1 cup water
- 1 tbsp Worcestershire sauce
- 1 tsp Italian seasoning
- ¾ tsp salt
- ½ tsp garlic powder
- 8 oz whole-wheat rotini or fusilli
- ½ cup shredded extra-sharp Cheddar cheese
- ¼ cup chopped fresh basil for garnish

**Directions:**

1. Heat oil in a large skillet over medium heat.
2. Add beef, mushrooms and onion and cook, stirring, until the beef is no longer pink and the mushroom liquid has mostly evaporated (8 to 10 minutes)
3. Stir in tomato sauce, water, Worcestershire, Italian seasoning, salt and garlic powder.
4. Add pasta. Bring to a boil.
5. Cover, reduce heat and cook, stirring once or twice, until the pasta is tender and most of the liquid is absorbed (16 to 18 minutes)
6. Sprinkle the pasta with cheese, cover and cook until the cheese is melted (2 to 3 minutes)
7. Garnish with basil, if desired.

## Honey-Garlic Chicken with Carrots and Broccoli

This sweet and savory baked honey-garlic chicken recipe with a side of veggies that cook in one pan is perfect for the weeknight dinner.

**Time:** 1 hour and 15 minutes
**Serving Size:** 2 chicken thighs and 1 cup veggies
**Servings Per Recipe**: 4
**Prep Time:** 55 minutes
**Cook Time:** 20 minutes
**Nutritional Facts:**

| Calories | 475kcal |
|----------|---------|
| Carbs | 40g |
| Fat | 20g |
| Protein | 36g |

### Ingredients:

- ⅓ cup honey
- 1 ½ tbsp reduced-sodium soy sauce
- 4 cloves garlic, minced (about 1 ½ tbsp)
- 1 tbsp cider vinegar
- ¼ tsp crushed red pepper
- 8 (5 oz) bone-in, skin-on chicken thighs
- 1 lbs small carrots, sliced into ½ -inch pieces
- 2 tbsp olive oil, divided

- 4 cups broccoli florets
- ½ tsp salt
- ½ tsp ground pepper
- 1 tsp cornstarch
- 1 tsp water

**Directions:**

1. Whisk honey, soy sauce, garlic, vinegar and crushed red pepper in a small bowl.
2. Place chicken and half of the honey mixture (about ¼ cup) in a zip-top plastic bag; remove excess air and seal the bag. Massage the chicken in the sealed bag until well coated.
3. Refrigerate for at least 30 minutes and up to 2 hours. Reserve the remaining honey mixture.
4. Preheat the oven to 400°F. Line a large rimmed baking sheet with foil; coat with cooking spray.
5. Remove the chicken from the marinade (discard marinade); arrange on 1 side of the prepared pan.
6. Combine carrots and 1 tablespoon oil in a medium bowl; toss well to coat. Spread the carrots in an even layer on the other side of the pan.
7. Bake the chicken and carrots for 15 minutes. Remove from the oven; stir the carrots.
8. Combine broccoli and the remaining 1 tablespoon oil; toss well to coat.
9. Distribute the broccoli evenly over the chicken and carrots on the pan. Sprinkle salt and pepper over all.
10. Bake until the vegetables are tender and a thermometer inserted in the thickest portion of the

chicken registers 165°F, 15 to 18 minutes.
11. Meanwhile, whisk cornstarch and water in a small bowl until no clumps remain.
12. Combine the cornstarch mixture and the reserved honey mixture in a small saucepan; bring to a simmer over medium-low heat, whisking once or twice.
13. Simmer, whisking often, until the sauce is clear and thickened, about 2 minutes.
14. Drizzle over the chicken and vegetables. Serve hot.

**Chicken Shawarma Bowls**

Savor a spiced chicken bowl with fresh veggies and tangy yogurt

**Time:** 1 hour and 25 minutes
**Serving Size:** 1 bowl
**Prep Time:** 25 minutes
**Cook Time:** 1 hour
**Nutritional Facts:**

| Calories | 730kcal |
|----------|---------|
| Carbs | 55g |
| Fat | 29g |
| Protein | 59g |

**Ingredients:**

Chicken:

- 1 tsp. ground cumin
- 1 tbsp. extra-virgin olive oil
- 1 tbsp. smoked paprika
- 2 tsp. ground coriander
- 1 ½ tsp. kosher salt
- ½ tsp. ground turmeric
- ¼ tsp. cayenne pepper
- ¼ tsp. ground cinnamon
- Freshly ground black pepper
- 2 lb. boneless, skinless chicken thighs

Bowls:

- 1 cup long-grain white rice, rinsed, drained
- Kosher salt
- 1 ½ tbsp. extra-virgin olive oil
- 2 small cucumbers, sliced into half-moons
- 2 bell peppers, chopped
- 1/4 red onion, thinly sliced
- 1 cup cherry tomatoes, halved
- ½ cup crumbled feta
- Pinch of crushed red pepper flakes
- Juice of 2 lemons, divided
- 1 cup plain Greek yogurt
- 1 tbsp. chopped fresh dill
- Store-bought or homemade hummus and pita(optional)

**Directions:**

1. In a medium pot over medium heat, combine rice, a large pinch of salt, and 2 cups of water. Bring to a boil.
2. Reduce heat to low, cover, and cook until rice is tender, about 15 minutes.
3. Remove from heat and keep covered, 10 minutes, then fluff rice with a fork.
4. Meanwhile, in a large skillet over medium-high heat, heat 1 tablespoon of oil.
5. Cook seasoned chicken, turning occasionally, until golden brown about 7 minutes per side.
6. Transfer chicken to a cutting board and let rest for 10 minutes, then slice into thin strips.
7. In a large bowl, combine cucumbers, bell peppers, onion, tomatoes, and feta.
8. Add red pepper, juice from 1 lemon, and remaining 2 teaspoons oil; season with salt. Toss to combine.
9. In a small bowl, stir yogurt, dill, and juice from the remaining 1 lemon.
10. Divide rice among bowls. Top with chicken, veggies, a dollop of yogurt sauce, and a dollop of hummus. Serve with pita alongside.

## One-pot Chicken Parmesan Pasta

This is a one-pot meal that comes together at the end, bringing the flavors of each ingredient to life.

**Time:** 35 minutes
**Serving Size:** 1½ cups
**Servings Per Recipe**: 4
**Prep Time:** 10 minutes
**Cook Time:** 35 minutes
**Nutritional Facts:**

| Calories | 538kcal |
|----------|---------|
| Carbs | 56g |
| Fat | 17g |
| Protein | 41g |

**Ingredients:**

- 2 tablespoons extra-virgin olive oil, divided
- ¼ cup whole-wheat panko breadcrumbs
- 1 tablespoon plus 1 teaspoon minced garlic, divided
- 1 pound boneless, skinless chicken breast, cubed
- 1 teaspoon Italian seasoning
- ¼ teaspoon salt
- 3 cups low-sodium chicken broth
- 1 ½ cups crushed tomatoes
- 8 ounces whole-wheat penne

- ½ cup shredded mozzarella cheese
- ¼ cup shredded Parmesan cheese
- ¼ cup chopped fresh basil

**Directions:**

1. Heat 1 tablespoon of oil in a large skillet over medium-high heat.
2. Add panko and 1 teaspoon garlic. Cook, stirring, until the panko is golden brown, (1 to 2 minutes) Transfer to a small bowl and set aside. Wipe out the pan.
3. Heat the remaining 1 tablespoon oil in the pan over medium-high heat.
4. Add chicken, Italian seasoning, salt and the remaining 1 tablespoon garlic.
5. Cook, stirring frequently, until the chicken is no longer pink on the outside, about 2 minutes.
6. Add broth, tomatoes and penne. Bring to a boil and cook, uncovered, stirring frequently, until the penne is cooked and the sauce has reduced and thickened, about 15 to 20 minutes.
7. Meanwhile, position an oven rack in the upper third of the oven. Preheat the broiler to 450°F..
8. When the pasta is cooked, sprinkle mozzarella over the penne mixture.
9. Place the pan under the broiler; broil until the mozzarella is bubbling and beginning to brown, about 1 minute.
10. Top with the panko mixture, Parmesan and basil.

## 10 Healthy Snacks

### Homemade Mozzarella Sticks (Air fried)

Enjoy your favorite crispy, cheesy appetizers without the guilt.

**Time:** 1 hour and 30 minutes
**Serving Size:** 4 sticks
**Servings Per Recipe:** 4
**Prep Time:** 20 minutes
**Cook Time:** 10 mins
**Chill time:** 1 Hour
**Nutritional Facts:**

| Calories | 323 kcal |
|----------|----------|
| Carbs | 27g |
| Fat | 14g |
| Protein | 20g |

**Ingredients:**

- 8 mozzarella string cheese sticks
- 3 large eggs
- 1 tbsp. water
- ½ cup. breadcrumbs
- ½ cup panko breadcrumbs
- 1 tsp. Italian seasoning blend

- ¼ tsp. garlic powder
- ¼ tsp. smoked paprika
- ⅓ cup all-purpose flour
- ½ tsp. salt
- ¼ tsp. ground black pepper
- Nonstick cooking spray
- Marinara sauce, to serve

**Directions:**

1. Cut the cheese sticks in half.
2. Whisk together the eggs and water in a bowl.
3. In another bowl, mix the breadcrumbs, panko, Italian seasoning, garlic powder, and smoked paprika.
4. In a third bowl, mix the flour, salt, and pepper.
5. Dip each of the cheese sticks into the egg mixture, then coat in the flour mixture pressing firmly. Repeat.
6. Place the coated sticks on a parchment-lined baking sheet. Freeze for 30 minutes.
7. After 30 minutes, dip each of the cheese sticks into the egg mixture, then coat in the breadcrumb mixture.
8. Freeze for another 30 minutes.
9. Preheat the air fryer to 390° F. Generously coat the frozen sticks with cooking spray.
10. Place the sticks in the basket in a single layer. Cook for 6 to 7 minutes or until browned and crispy. (Keep an eye on them so the cheese dosent start to bubble out.)
11. Serve immediately with warm marinara sauce.

## Homemade Granola Bars

The perfect balance of nutritious ingredients and irresistible flavor. These chewy granola bars are the perfect morning or afternoon snack on the go.

**Time:** 2 hours and 20 minutes
**Serving Size:** 1 bar
**Servings Per Recipe:** 10
**Prep Time:** 10 minutes
**Cook Time:** 10 minutes
**Chill time:** 2 hours minimum
**Nutritional Facts:**

| Calories | 260kcal |
|----------|---------|
| Carbs    | 39g     |
| Fat      | 11g     |
| Protein  | 5g      |

Ingredients:

- ½ cups old fashioned rolled oats
- ½ cup whole almonds, roughly chopped
- ⅓ cup honey
- ¼ cup unsalted butter
- ¼ cup dark brown sugar
- 1 tsp vanilla extract
- 1 tsp chia seeds

- ¼ tsp kosher salt
- ¼ cup dried cranberries
- ¼ cup dried golden raisins
- ¼ cup mini chocolate chips, plus extra as needed

**Directions:**

1. Heat oven to 350°F . Line the bottom of a 9-inch square pan with parchment paper. Lightly spray the parchment with cooking spray.
2. Add the oats and roughly chopped almonds to a small baking sheet then bake for 10 minutes until lightly toasted. Transfer to a large bowl.
3. While the oats are toasting, mix the butter, honey, brown sugar, vanilla extract seeds, chia and salt in a saucepan over medium heat. Cook until melted and make sure to stir occasionally.
4. Pour the butter mixture over the toasted oats and almonds and add the cranberries and golden raisins. Mix it well.
5. Let cool for 15 minutes then add the mini chocolate chips and mix again.
6. Transfer the oat mixture to the prepared pan. Firmly press the mixture into the pan until the mixture is in an even layer.
7. Scatter remaining a few extra tablespoons of mini chocolate chips on top and press gently into the granola so they stick.
8. Transfer the entire pan to the refrigerator and chill for at least 2 hours.

9. Once it's cooled completely, carefully lift it out of the pan using the parchment paper and cut it into the desired shape.

### Strawberry Banana Smoothie

Filling and tasty smoothie that will only take 5 minutes of your time.

**Time:** 5 minutes
**Serving Size:** 12oz
**Serving Per Recipe:** 2
**Prep Time:** 5 minutes
**Cook Time:** No cooking Required!
**Nutritional Facts:**

| Calories | 211kcal |
|----------|---------|
| Carbs | 42g |
| Fat | 4g |
| Protein | 7g |

**Ingredients:**

- 1 ¼ cups milk
- 2 cups frozen strawberries
- 1 frozen banana
- 1 Tbsp ground flaxseed , or chia seeds
- 1-2 Tbsp honey

**Directions:**

- Add the milk, strawberries, banana, flaxseed and honey in a blender.
- Blend until smooth and creamy.

### Kale Chips (Air fried)

Indulge guilt-free with this delicious and healthy alternative to satisfy chip cravings!

**Time:** 10 minutes
**Serving Size:** 3oz
**Serving Per Recipe:** 4
**Prep Time:** 5 minutes
**Cook Time:** 5 minutes
**Nutritional Facts:**

| Calories | 154kcal |
|----------|---------|
| Carbs | 2g |
| Fat | 12g |
| Protein | 8g |

**Ingredients:**

- 1 bunch kale washed and dried
- 2 tbsp. extra-virgin olive oil
- 1 tbsp. fresh lemon juice

- ½ cup finely grated Parmesan
- Kosher salt and Freshly ground black pepper
- Optional seasonings: everything bagel seasoning, smoked paprika, crushed red pepper flakes, or garlic powder

**Directions:**

1. Tear kale leaves into large pieces and transfer to a medium bowl.
2. Drizzle with oil and lemon juice and toss using your fingers to ensure each piece is lightly and evenly coated.
3. Add Parmesan, season with salt and black pepper and any optional seasonings to taste. Toss again to combine.
4. In an air-fryer basket, arrange kale in a single layer. Cook at 350°F until the edges are just starting to brown (3 to 5 minutes).
5. Transfer kale to a sheet pan and let cool in a single layer. The kale will crisp as it cools!

**Fruit Salad**

Bursting with flavors, this is a refreshing treat for any occasion.

**Time:** 10 minutes
**Serving Size:** 4oz
**Serving Per Recipe:** 4
**Prep Time:** 10 minutes

**Cook Time:** No cooking Required!
**Nutritional Facts:**

| Calories | 283kcal |
|----------|---------|
| Carbs | 72g |
| Fat | 1g |
| Protein | 3g |

**Ingredients:**

- ½ lb fresh strawberry, quartered
- 2 kiwis, peeled and diced
- 2 mangoes, diced
- 2 bananas, sliced
- ½ lb fresh blueberry
- 2 tablespoons honey
- 1 lime, juiced

**Directions:**

1. Combine sliced fruits in a large bowl.
2. In a small bowl, mix honey and lime juice.
3. Pour syrup over the fruit and mix.

## Edamame Beans

Indulge in a delightful and nutritious treat with Edemmame: Packed with protein, fiber, and essential nutrients, it's a guilt-free snack or side that's as wholesome as it is delicious.

**Time:** 20 minutes
**Serving Size:** 2.5 oz
**Servings Per Recipe:** 6
**Prep Time:** 5 minutes
**Cook Time:** 15 minutes
**Nutritional Facts:**

| Calories | 60kcal |
|----------|--------|
| Carb | 4g |
| Fat | 3g |
| Protein | 5g |

**Ingredients:**

Chicken Salt:

- 2 boullion cubes
- 2 tsp. garlic powder
- 2 tsp. onion powder
- ½ tsp. celery salt
- ½ tsp. smoked paprika
- ¼ tsp. MSG (optional)

- ¼ tsp. turmeric

Edammame:

- Kosher salt
- 1 lb. fresh or frozen edamame

**Directions:**

1. In a small bowl, crush bouillon cubes into a powder. Add garlic powder, onion powder, celery salt, paprika, MSG, and turmeric.
2. Mix until thoroughly combined. Make Ahead: Salt can be made 6 months ahead. Store in an airtight container at room temperature.
3. Meanwhile, in a large pot, pour water to a depth of about ½ inch. Stir in 2 teaspoons of kosher salt, then bring to a boil.
4. In a steam basket, place edamame and lower into pot. Cover and steam until beans are fully tender, 8 to 10 minutes. It may take longer if frozen.
5. Drain beans and transfer to a large bowl. Add 1 teaspoon chicken salt, season with kosher salt, and toss well to combine.

## Crunchy Chilli Chickpeas (Air Fried)

Zesty chickpeas, a dash of chili, lime zest; Biting into these will cure your addiction to any other food!

**Time:** 20 minutes
**Serving Size:** 4oz
**Serving Per Recipe:** 4
**Prep Time:** 5 minutes
**Cook Time:** 15minutes
**Nutritional Facts:**

| Calories | 182kcal |
|----------|---------|
| Carbs    | 17g     |
| Fat      | 7g      |
| Protein  | 8g      |

## Ingredients:

- 1 (15-oz.) can chickpeas, rinsed and drained
- 1 tbsp. extra-virgin olive oil
- 2 tsp. chili powder
- 1/4 tsp. kosher salt
- Finely grated lime zest, for garnish

**Directions:**

1. Dry chickpeas very well with paper towels.
2. In a medium bowl, toss chickpeas, oil, chili powder, and salt.
3. Transfer chickpea mixture to an air-fryer basket,Cook at 370° until crispy and golden brown, 10 to 14 minutes.
4. Grate lime zest over top.

### Lemon Garlic Roated Broccoli

Vibrant broccoli meets zesty lemon for a wholesome, healthy treat.

**Time:** 20 minutes
**Serving Size:** 1 (136 g)
**Servings Per Recipe**: 4
**Prep Time:** 5 minutes
**Cook Time:** 15 minutes
**Nutritional Facts:**

| Calories | 172kcal |
|----------|---------|
| Carbs | 7g |
| Fat | 16g |
| Protein | 4g |

**Ingredients:**

- 1lbs broccoli floret
- 2 tbsp olive oil
- salt & freshly ground black pepper
- 2 tbsp unsalted butter
- 1 tsp garlic, minced
- ½ tsp lemon zest, grated
- 1 -2 tbsp fresh lemon juice
- 2 tbsp pine nuts, toasted

**Directions:**

1. Preheat the oven to 500 °F .
2. Toss the broccoli with the oil and salt and pepper to taste in a large bowl.
3. Spred the florets in a single layer on a baking sheet and roast for 12 minutes, turning once halfway through
4. Meanwhile, melt the butter over medium heat in a small pan.
5. Add the garlic and lemon zest, stirring, for about 1 minute.
6. Let cool slightly and mix in the lemon juice.
7. Place the broccoli in a serving bowl, pour the lemon butter over it and toss to coat.
8. Top with toasted pine nuts

## Caramelized Cauliflower Popcorn

Caramelized cauliflower—a delightful, healthy treat!

**Time:** 1 hour 10 minutes
**Serving Size:** 1 (62 g)
**Servings Per Recipe**: 4
**Prep Time:** 10 minutes
**Cook Time:** 1 hour
**Nutritional Facts:**

| Calories | 156kcal |
|----------|---------|
| Carbs | 7g |
| Fat | 14g |
| Protein | 3g |

**Ingredients:**

- 1 head cauliflower
- 4 tbsp olive oil
- 1 tsp salt, to taste

**Directions:**

1. Preheat the oven to 425 °F.
2. Trim the head of the cauliflower, discarding the core and thick stems; cut florets into pieces

3. In a large bowl, mix the olive oil and salt, whisk, then add the cauliflower florets and toss thoroughly.
4. Spread evenly on a sheet pan and roast for 1 hour, turning 3 or 4 times, each piece is mostly golden brown.

### Crispy Bacon and Brussels Sprouts

Brussels sprouts: now starring in a savory bacon and onion symphony!

**Time:** 20 minutes
**Serving Size**: 1 (123 g)
**Servings Per Recipe**: 6
**Prep Time:** 5 minutes
**Cook Time:** 15 minutes
**Nutritional Facts:**

| Calories | 45kcal |
|----------|--------|
| Carbs | 7g |
| Fat | 14g |
| Protein | 2g |

**Ingredients:**

- 2 slices bacon
- 1 small yellow onion, thinly sliced
- ¼ tsp salt (or to taste)

- ¾ cup water
- 1 tsp Dijon mustard
- 1 lb Brussels sprout, thinly sliced
- 1 tbsp cider vinegar

**Directions:**

1. Cook bacon in high heat until crispy.
2. Drain on paper and crumble, but don't discard the oil.
3. In the bacon oil, add the onion and salt. Cook until the onion is slightly brown but not dark.
4. Add the mustard, and water to deglaze the pan.
5. Add the brussel sprouts and cook until tender.
6. Stir in the vinegar and top with the crumbled bacon.

*10 Guilt-Free Desserts*

### Chocolate Covered Banana Bites

Delightful chocolate-covered bananas for a satisfying and guilt-free treat.

**Time:** 8 hours and 10 mins
**Serving Size:** 4 bites
**Servings Per Recipe:** 5
**Prep Time:** 10 minutes
**Cook/chill Time:** 8 hours (overnight)

## Nutritional Facts:

| Calories | 180kcal |
|----------|---------|
| Carbs | 15g |
| Fat | 14g |
| Protein | 1g |

## Ingredients:

- 2 ripe bananas
- 5 tbsp coconut oil (melted)
- 3-4 tbsp unsweetened cocoa powder

## Directions:

1. Cut bananas into thin slices.
2. Place on a tray lined with parchment paper and pop into the freezer overnight or until frozen.
3. Meanwhile, mix the coconut oil and cocoa together until thick enough to stick to the bananas
4. One by one, dip the frozen bananas into the chocolate mixture.
5. Pop the coated bananas back onto the tray and into the freezer for another 15 minutes to ensure they have fully set.

## Strawberry Crumble

Strawberry crumble, a dessert that is healthful and easy to make!

**Time:** 45 minutes
**Serving Size:** 1 (263g)
**Serving Per Recipe:** 4
**Prep Time:** 15 minutes
**Cook:** 30 minutes
**Nutritional Facts:**

| Calories | 336kcal |
|----------|---------|
| Carbs | 35g |
| Fat | 25g |
| Protein | 7g |

**Ingredients:**

- 4 cups strawberries halved
- 2 tbsp tapioca starch
- 2 tsp vanilla extract
- 1 tbsp fresh lemon juice
- 1 tbsp pure maple syrup

For the crumble topping:

- 1 cup almond meal/flour
- ½ tsp kosher salt
- 3 tsp coconut oil or grapeseed oil
- 3 tbsp pure maple syrup

**Directions:**

1. Preheat the oven to 350 °F.
2. Meanwhile, In a mixing bowl, toss together the strawberries, tapioca starch, vanilla extract, lemon juice, and maple syrup.
3. Transfer mixture to an 8" x 8" baking pan.
4. Mix together the ingredients for the crumble topping in a mixing bowl.
5. Evenly spread it over the strawberries and bake in the oven for 30 minutes, until the strawberries are juicy and bubbly and the topping is golden-brown.
6. Let stand for 10 minutes before serving.

### Chocolate Chip Energy Bites

Enjoy an energy boost after a workout or any time you feel like a quick, sweet treat!

**Time:** 2 hours and 10 minutes
**Serving Size:** 1 ball
**Servings Per Recipe:** 20
**Prep Time:** 10 minutes
**Cook time:** No cooking required!

**Chill time** 2 hours
**Nutritional Facts:**

| Calories | 193kcal |
|----------|---------|
| Carbs | 19g |
| Fat | 12g |
| Protein | 5g |

**Ingredients:**

- 1 cup rolled oats
- 2/3 cup shredded coconut (toasted)
- 1/2 cup smooth peanut butter
- 1 1/2 cup flax seed (ground)
- 1/2 cup dark chocolate chips
- 1/3 cup honey
- 1 tsp vanilla extract

**Directions:**

1. Combine all ingredients in a large bowl.
2. Chill for 1–2 hours (not overnight).
3. With the palm of your hand, roll the mixture into 1-inch balls.

## Honey Roasted Peaches

These delightful treats are sufficiently tangy and airy to serve as a breakfast option, yet they possess enough sweetness and indulgence to also be enjoyed as a guilt-free dessert.

**Time:** 30 minutes
**Serving Size:** ½ peach
**Servings Per Recipe:** 4
**Prep Time:** 5 minutes
**Cook Time:** 25 minutes
**Nutritional Facts:**

| Calories | 158kcal |
|----------|---------|
| Carbs | 26g |
| Fat | 3g |
| Protein | 9g |

**Ingredients:**

- 2 Large ripe peaches
- 2 tbsp light butter
- ½ tsp ground cinnamon
- 2 tbsp honey
- 12oz fat-free vanilla Greek yogurt

**Directions:**

1. Preheat the oven to 350 °F.
2. Cut the peaches in half and remove the stone.
3. On each peach half, add 1/2 tbsp of butter, ½ tbsp of honey, and top with a sprinkle of cinnamon.
4. Bake for 20–30 minutes until the peaches are soft and the edges are browning.
5. Allow to cool before serving with 3oz of yogurt..

### Banana Coconut Muffins

A delicious and nutritious treat, perfect for satisfying your sweet cravings while nourishing your body.

**Time:** 45 minutes
**Serving Size:** 1 muffin
**Serving Per Recipe:** 12
**Prep Time:** 15 minutes
**Cook Time:** 30 minutes
**Nutritional Facts:**

| Calories | 300kcal |
|----------|---------|
| Carbs | 40g |
| Fat | 15g |
| Protein | 3g |

**Ingredients:**

- 2 cups all-purpose flour
- 1 cup granulated sugar
- 1 cup unsweetened dried shredded coconut
- 2 teaspoons baking soda
- 1 teaspoon baking powder
- ½ teaspoon salt
- 2 ripe bananas, mashed
- 1 ½ cups coconut milk
- ¼ cup cold-pressed liquid coconut oil
- 1 teaspoon vanilla extract

**Directions:**

1. Preheat the oven to 350°F (180°C). Spray 12-count muffin tray with cooking spray. Set aside.
2. Meanwhile, whisk together flour, sugar, coconut, baking soda, baking powder and salt in a large bowl. Set aside.
3. Mix together bananas, kefir, coconut oil and vanilla in a separate large bowl.
4. Add to flour mixture; stir until no white streaks remain.
5. Divide among the wells of the prepared muffin tray.
6. Bake for about 30 minutes.
7. Let cool in a muffin tray for 15 minutes.

## Strawberry and Rhubarb Parfait

Roasted strawberries and rhubarb, sweetened with honey, create a deliciously tangy sauce.

**Time:** 30 minutes
**Serving Size:** 3oz
**Serving Per Recipe:** 4
**Prep Time:** 10 minutes
**Cook Time:** 20 minutes
**Nutritional Facts:** *(Sauce only)*

| Calories | 144kcal |
|----------|---------|
| Carbs | 37g |
| Fat | 0.5g |
| Protein | 2g |

**Ingredients:**

- 2 1/2 cups strawberries (hulled and sliced)
- 2 1/2 cups rhubarb (cut into 1/4-inch wide slices)
- 1/3 cup honey
- 1 small lemon (juiced)

Parfait:

- Granola(optional)
- 32 ounces plain yogurt (Greek yogurt/vanilla yogurt works, too)

**Directions:**

1. Preheat the oven to 350 °F.
2. In a single layer, add the strawberry and rhubarb pieces tossed in honey to a lined baking tray.
3. Bake for 25 minutes. Toss again halfway.
4. Once the fruit is cooked, add the pieces to a bowl and stir in the lemon juice.
5. In small glasses or bowls, layer yogurt, strawberry-rhubarb sauce and granola as desired.

### Spicy Chocolate Cups

These decadent dark chocolate treats are infused with a hint of cinnamon, complemented by toasted coconut flakes and a touch of cayenne for a spicy twist.

**Time:** 40 minutes
**Serving Size:** 1 muffin
**Servings Per Recipe:** 24
**Prep Time:** 10 minutes
**Cook Time:** 30 minutes

**Nutritional Facts:**

| Calories | 110kcal |
|----------|---------|
| Carbs | 4g |
| Fat | 10g |
| Protein | 2g |

**Ingredients:**

- ⅔ cup coconut oil
- ⅔ cup smooth peanut butter
- ½ cup dark cocoa
- 4 packets stevia (or to taste)
- 1 tbsp ground cinnamon
- ¼ tsp kosher salt
- ½ cup toasted coconut flakes
- ¼ tsp cayenne (to taste)

**Directions:**

1. Combine coconut oil, peanut butter, and cocoa powder and set over a pot of simmering water. Heat, stirring, until melted and smooth.
2. Add stevia, cinnamon, and salt and stir to combine.
3. Divide mixture among a silicone mini muffin tray.
4. Top with coconut and cayenne and transfer to the freezer until firm, (about 30 minutes).

## Homemade Chocolate Truffles

This could be a take on the classic banana bread, or it could be something new entirely.

**Time:** 30 minutes
**Serving Size:** 2 truffles
**Servings Per Recipe:** 5
**Prep Time:** 10 minutes
**Chill Time:** 20 minutes
**Nutritional Facts:**

| Calories | 110kcal |
|----------|---------|
| Carbs | 9g |
| Fat | 7g |
| Protein | 2.5g |

**Ingredients:**

- ½ cup good quality chocolate chips (at least 60 % cocoa)
- 1 tbsp all natural almond butter, peanut butter or any other nut butter
- ¼ cup fat free Greek yogurt
- 1 tbsp unsweetened cocoa powder

**Directions:**

1. Melt chocolate chips in the microwave (at 20 second intervals)
2. In a separate bowl, whisk together the Greek Yogurt and nut butter.
3. Add the melted chocolate and mix well.
4. Refrigerate until it starts to harden
5. Working with 2 tablespoons at a time form truffles,
6. Roll them in the unsweetened cocoa powder

**Chocolate Avacado and Peanut Butter Pudding**

Thick and creamy nutrient packed pudding.

**Time:** 3 hours and 10 Minutes
**Serving Size:** 1 cup
**Servings Per Recipe:** 6
**Prep Time:** 10 minutes
**Cook/chill Time:** 3 hours (minimum)
**Nutritional Facts:**

| Calories | 386kcal |
|----------|---------|
| Carbs | 29g |
| Fat | 29g |
| Protein | 9g |

## Ingredients:

- 1½ ripe avocados
- 1 large ripe banana
- ½ cup unsweetened cocoa or cacao powder
- ½ cup salted creamy or crunchy peanut butter (plus more for topping)
- ½ cup maple syrup or honey
- ¼ cup almond milk or other non-dairy milk

## Directions:

1. Combine all ingredients in a blender and mix..
2. Separate into six small cups or dessert bowls and cover with plastic wrap.
3. Place in the fridge and chill for a few hours, or overnight.

### Frozen Fruit Pops

Enjoy these fresh fruit pops on a hot summer day.

**Time:** 11 hours and 15 minutes
**Serving Size:** 1 pop
**Servings Per Recipe:** 4
**Prep Time:** 10 minutes
**Cook Time:** 5 minutes
**Chill Time:** 11 hours

**Nutritional Facts:**

| Calories | 91kcal |
|----------|--------|
| Carbs | 22g |
| Fat | 0.5g |
| Protein | 1g |

**Ingredients:**

- 9 tbsp water
- 2 tbsp sugar
- 5 oz kiwi, peeled
- 6 oz mango, peeled
- 6 oz fresh raspberries

**Directions:**

1. Combine water and sugar in a small pot and bring to a boil; boil for about 4-5 minutes on medium heat making a simple syrup and Set aside.
2. Puree each fruit separately in the blender. Set aside in 3 small bowls.
3. Divide the simple syrup between the fruit purees and mix in.
4. Equally fill four small 5 oz cups with the kiwi puree and place in the freezer; freeze for one hour.
5. Then add mango puree over the kiwi and freeze for another 20 minutes.

6. Insert sticks and freeze for at least 2 more hours.
7. Lastly, add raspberry puree on top and freeze overnight.

❄

## Exploring Unique Benefits

Each type of meal in our collection offers unique benefits tailored to the needs of women over 50. Here's a closer look at why these meals are specifically suitable for supporting hormonal balance and overall well-being:

1. **Protein-Packed Breakfasts:** Starting your day with a protein-rich breakfast provides sustained energy to fuel your morning activities. Protein helps stabilize blood sugar levels and promotes feelings of fullness, reducing the likelihood of overeating later in the day. For women over 50, maintaining muscle mass becomes increasingly essential, and protein-packed breakfasts support muscle maintenance and repair.

2. **Light Dinners:** Lighter dinners promote easier digestion and may improve sleep quality. Heavy meals before bedtime can disrupt sleep patterns and lead to indigestion, which can be exceptionally bothersome for women experiencing hormonal fluctuations during menopause. Light dinners focus on lean proteins, vegetables, and whole grains, providing essential nutrients without weighing you down.

3. **Fiber-Rich Lunches:** Incorporating fiber-rich foods into your midday meal supports digestive health and helps regulate blood sugar levels. Fiber promotes satiety and aids in weight management by boosting feelings of fullness. Additionally, fiber-rich lunches can help alleviate constipation, a common issue for women over 50, and support overall gut health.

4. **Healthy Snacks:** Snacking can be essential for maintaining energy levels and preventing overeating during intermittent fasting. Healthy snacks provide a convenient way to satisfy hunger between meals without derailing your fasting goals. Opt for nutrient-dense snacks like nuts, seeds, Greek yogurt, or fresh fruit to keep you satisfied and energized throughout the day.

## 7-Day Meal Plan

Now, let's put these principles into action with a 7-day meal plan designed to support hormonal balance and overall health for women over 50:

**Day 1:**

- **Breakfast:** Blueberry Pecan Overnight Oats
- **Lunch:** Greek Salad Wrap
- **Dinner:** Lemon Garlic Chicken Pasta
- **Snack:** Kale Chips (Air fried)

**Day 2:**

- **Breakfast:** Poached Egg on Avocado Toast
- **Lunch:** Black Bean Soup
- **Dinner:** Rosemary Walnut Crusted Salmon
- **Snack:** Homemade Granola Bars

**Day 3:**

- **Breakfast:** Tropical Acai Bowl
- **Lunch:** Veggie Delight Sandwich
- **Dinner:** Honey-Garlic Chicken with Carrots and Broccoli
- **Snack:** Fruit Salad

**Day 4:**

- **Breakfast:** Chocolate Quinoa Bowl
- **Lunch:** Shrimp and Soba Noodle Salad
- **Dinner:** Sheet Pan Chicken Fajitas
- **Snack:** Edamame Beans

**Day 5:**

- **Breakfast:** Greek Yogurt and Berry Bowl
- **Lunch:** Sauerkraut Salad
- **Dinner:** Beef & Mushroom Pasta Skillet
- **Snack:** Crunchy Chilli Chickpeas (Air Fried)

**Day 6:**

- **Breakfast:** Buttered Apple Muffins
- **Lunch:** Greek Salad Wrap
- **Dinner:** Chicken Shawarma Bowls
- **Snack:** Lemon Garlic Roasted Broccoli

**Day 7:**

- **Breakfast:** Shakshuka with Greens
- **Lunch:** Cheesy Chicken Salad
- **Dinner:** One-pot Chicken Parmesan Pasta
- **Snack:** Caramelized Cauliflower Popcorn

Feel free to adjust portion sizes and ingredients according to your preferences and dietary requirements. Enjoy your meals!

## Tips for Modification

While our meal plan provides a comprehensive guide to balanced eating, it's essential to customize recipes to meet individual nutritional needs and preferences. Here are some tips for modifying recipes:

- Swap ingredients to accommodate dietary restrictions or preferences. For example, use tofu or tempeh for plant-based protein options instead of meat.
- Adjust portion sizes to align with calorie and macronutrient goals. For women over 50, portion control is key to maintaining a healthy weight and supporting hormonal balance.

- Experiment with different flavor combinations and cooking methods to keep meals exciting and enjoyable. Adding herbs, spices, and healthy fats can enhance dishes' taste and nutritional profile.

This chapter explores the importance of a balanced diet in supporting hormonal health for women over 50. You can optimize hormonal balance and overall well-being by incorporating nutrient-rich foods and mindful meal timing into your intermittent fasting regimen. However, diet is just one piece of the puzzle. In the next chapter, we'll focus on the other crucial component of a healthy lifestyle—exercise routines designed for women over 50. Stay tuned as we continue our journey toward vibrant health and vitality.

FOUR

# Routines in Exercise

To exercise is to be healthy, and being healthy is easier when you exercise. Intermittent fasting is the first step to a healthier, happier you. If you combine this with exercise, your transition will be as radiant and as full of life as you are. The building blocks of a healthy lifestyle combine exercise and diet into a single movement. As we age, this becomes more important but can also feel more difficult. With the right tools and mindset, we can synergize the relationship between intermittent fasting and exercise with willpower and perseverance.

In this chapter, we'll delve into the importance of exercise at this stage in life, explore various exercises suitable for women over 50, and discuss how exercise complements intermittent fasting for weight loss and energy gain. We'll also provide practical guidance for creating a simple and effective exercise routine tailored to your needs.

## Benefits of Exercise for Women Over 50

As women age, reaching the milestone of 50 and beyond, maintaining a regular exercise routine becomes increasingly crucial. This period brings about significant changes in the body, both physically and hormonally, making exercise an essential component for overall health and well-being.

One of the primary reasons why exercise is particularly crucial for women over 50 is its role in maintaining bone density. As women age, they become more susceptible to osteoporosis, a condition characterized by weakened bones prone to fractures. Research published in the Journal of Bone and Mineral Research found that postmenopausal women who engaged in regular weight-bearing exercises experienced less bone loss than sedentary women. Regular weight-bearing exercises like walking, jogging, or resistance training help stimulate bone growth and density, reducing the risk of osteoporosis and fractures. Women can preserve their bone health and maintain mobility and independence as they age by engaging in these activities.

Furthermore, exercise is vital in hormone regulation, especially during menopause. As women enter menopause, their estrogen levels decline, leading to various symptoms like hot flashes, mood swings, and weight gain. Exercise helps mitigate these symptoms by promoting the release of endorphins, the body's natural mood elevators, which can alleviate mood swings and reduce stress and anxiety associated with menopause. Additionally, regular physical activity can help manage weight gain by boosting metabolism and preserving lean muscle mass, which tends to decrease with age and hormonal changes.

Exercise offers numerous other benefits beyond bone health and hormone regulation. It helps improve cardiovascular health by reducing the risk of heart disease, stroke, and high blood pressure. A study published in the Journal of the American Heart Association revealed that engaging in moderate-intensity aerobic exercises, such as swimming or cycling, for at least 150 minutes per week can lower the risk of cardiovascular disease in women over 50 by up to 30%. Additionally, strength training exercises enhance muscle strength and endurance, promoting better balance and reducing the risk of falls and injuries, which becomes increasingly important as women age.

Moreover, exercise is crucial in maintaining cognitive function and mental well-being. Research cited by Livestrong indicates that regular exercise significantly benefits older adults' mental health and cognitive function. A study published in the British Journal of Sports Medicine found that women over 50 who engaged in regular physical activity experienced improvements in mood, memory, and overall cognitive function compared to their sedentary counterparts. Furthermore, the release of endorphins during exercise helps alleviate symptoms of depression and anxiety, as reported by WebMD.

Exercise, particularly strength training, enhances functional independence. According to Cone Health, strength training exercises help maintain muscle mass and strength, improve balance, and reduce the risk of falls and injuries. A study published in the Journal of the American Geriatrics Society found that older adults who participated in a strength training program experienced significant improvements in muscle strength, mobility, and functional independence.

Lastly, exercise is associated with increased longevity and reduced risk of premature death among older adults. Seniors.com.au cites a study published in the BMJ Open Sport & Exercise Medicine, which found that regular exercise can help women live longer, healthier lives. As recommended by the World Health Organization, engaging in physical activity for at least 150 minutes per week can contribute to longevity and overall well-being.

Incorporating exercise into daily life can seem daunting, especially for women with busy schedules or physical limitations. However, it's essential to find activities that are enjoyable and sustainable. Whether taking a brisk walk in the park, attending a yoga class, or dancing to your favorite music at home, there are countless ways to stay active and reap the benefits of exercise. It's always the right time to start reaping the rewards of regular physical activity, and by prioritizing exercise, we can enhance our health, vitality, and quality of life for years to come.

If the scientific data wasn't enough to convince you, here is what other women just like you have to say:

Sarah, a vibrant woman in her early 60s, discovered the transformative power of exercise later in life. After struggling with osteoporosis and feeling a loss of independence, Sarah decided to take charge of her health by incorporating regular strength training into her routine. With guidance from her trainer and dedication to her workouts, Sarah regained bone density and experienced newfound confidence and vitality. "I never thought I'd be lifting weights at my age," Sarah shares with a smile, "but now, I feel stronger and more capable than ever before. Exercise has given me back my freedom."

And then there's Priscilla, a vibrant woman over 50 who defied stereotypes and embraced a fitness journey that transformed her body and mind. Priscilla prioritized her well-being by committing to regular exercise sessions after facing health setbacks and feeling discouraged about her physical abilities. Priscilla felt her strength and confidence grow with each workout, and she soon achieved milestones she never thought possible. "Exercise has become my fountain of youth," Priscilla shares enthusiastically, "I feel healthier, happier, and more alive than ever. Age is just a number, and I refuse to let it define me."

These anecdotes illustrate the real-life impact of exercise on women, showcasing how regular physical activity can improve physical health, mental well-being, and overall quality of life. Through dedication, perseverance, and the support of a fitness community, Sarah, Priscilla, and countless others have redefined what it means to age gracefully and live life to the fullest.

## Exercises Suitable for You

Not all exercises are equal, especially for women over 50. As bodies change with age, choosing activities that address specific needs and promote overall well-being becomes crucial. Low-impact exercises like swimming or yoga can help maintain flexibility and joint health. At the same time, strength training preserves muscle mass and bone density. Tailoring workouts to individual fitness levels and goals ensures maximum benefits and minimizes the risk of injury.

**1. Walking**

Walking is one of the simplest yet most effective forms of exercise. It's low-impact, easy on the joints, and easily incorporated into daily life. Aim for at least 30 minutes of brisk walking most days of the week to reap its numerous health benefits, including improved cardiovascular health, weight management, and mood enhancement.

**2. Wall Pilates**

Wall Pilates is an excellent option for women over 50 looking to improve core strength, posture, and flexibility without putting undue stress on the joints. By using the wall for support, you can perform various Pilates exercises that target the core, upper body, and lower body muscles, helping to improve balance, stability, and overall body awareness.

## 3. Swimming

Swimming is a fantastic full-body workout that is gentle on the joints, making it ideal for women with arthritis or other joint issues. Whether you swim laps in the pool or take a water aerobics class, swimming can help improve cardiovascular fitness, muscle strength, and flexibility while providing a low-impact, enjoyable form of exercise.

## 4. Yoga

Yoga is another excellent option, offering many physical and mental benefits. Different styles of yoga, from gentle Hatha yoga to more vigorous Vinyasa flow, can be tailored to suit individual needs and preferences. Yoga improves flexibility, balance, strength, and mental well-being, making it an ideal exercise for promoting overall health and vitality.

## 5. Tai Chi

Tai Chi is a gentle martial art focusing on slow, flowing movements and deep breathing techniques. It's particularly beneficial for improving balance, coordination, and stress management. Tai Chi is an excellent exercise for women who want to improve their well-being while reducing the risk of falls and injuries.

## 6. Resistance Band Exercises

Resistance band exercises are a great way to build muscle strength and tone without heavy weights or gym equipment. Resistance bands come in various levels, making them suitable for all fitness levels. Incorporate resistance band exercises into your routine to target specific muscle groups and improve overall strength and stability.

### 7. Cycling

Cycling is an excellent low-impact exercise that can be easily tailored to individual fitness levels and preferences. Whether you prefer leisurely bike rides outdoors or high-intensity spin classes indoors, cycling can help improve cardiovascular fitness, leg strength, and overall endurance while being easy on the joints.

### 8. Weights

Strength training with weights is essential to help maintain muscle mass, bone density, and overall strength as we age. Start with light weights and gradually increase resistance as you build strength and confidence. To maximize efficiency and effectiveness, focus on compound exercises that target multiple muscle groups, such as squats, lunges, deadlifts, and chest presses.

### *How Exercise Complements Intermittent Fasting*

Exercise and intermittent fasting synergize to enhance weight loss, improve metabolic health, and increase energy levels. They create a powerful metabolic state that promotes fat burning, preserves lean muscle mass, and boosts overall metabolic rate. Additionally, exercise can help mitigate some of the potential side effects of intermittent fasting, such as hunger, fatigue, and irritability, by promoting the release of endorphins and improving mood and mental well-being.

Regarding exercise timing and type, it's essential to consider your fasting schedule and individual preferences. Some people may prefer to exercise in a fast state. In contrast, others may find it more comfortable to work out after breaking their fast. Experiment with different timings and types of exercise to see what works best for you and fits seamlessly into your intermittent fasting routine.

## Creating a Simple and Effective Exercise Routine

Exercise and intermittent fasting can synergize to produce better results, particularly in weight loss and energy gain, by leveraging the body's natural processes and optimizing metabolic function.

Intermittent fasting involves cycling between periods of eating and fasting, typically with daily fasting windows ranging from 12 to 20 hours. During fasting, the body depletes glycogen stores and relies on fat stores for energy. When combined with exercise, especially during fasting, the body becomes more efficient at burning fat for fuel. This process, known as fat adaptation, enhances weight loss by promoting fat metabolism and reducing reliance on glucose.

In addition to weight loss, exercise, and intermittent fasting can boost energy levels and cognitive function. Regular physical activity improves cardiovascular health, increases oxygen delivery to tissues, and enhances mitochondrial function, leading to greater energy production and stamina. Meanwhile, intermittent fasting promotes cellular repair and autophagy (cleansing damaged cells), which can improve brain function and mental clarity.

By integrating exercise and intermittent fasting into a holistic lifestyle, individuals can achieve effortless weight loss, increased energy levels, and improved metabolic health.

Here are some tips to create a simple and effective exercise routine tailored to you:

1. **Set realistic goals**: Start by defining your fitness goals, whether it's weight loss, muscle toning, improved flexibility, or overall health and well-being. Be specific, measurable, and realistic in setting your goals to ensure success.

2. **Choose activities you enjoy:** Find activities you enjoy and look forward to doing. Whether walking, swimming, yoga, or cycling, choose activities that fit your interests, preferences, and fitness level.

3. **Schedule regular workouts:** Consistency is key to success in any exercise routine. Schedule regular workouts into your weekly calendar and treat them as non-negotiable appointments with yourself.

4. **Start slowly and progress gradually:** If you're new to exercise or haven't been active, gradually increase the intensity, duration, and frequency of your workouts over time. Listen to your body, and don't push yourself too hard too soon to avoid injury or burnout.

5. **Incorporate variety:** Mix your workouts to prevent boredom, plateaus, and injuries. Include activities targeting different muscle groups and energy systems, such as cardio, strength training, flexibility exercises, and balance training.

**Monitor progress and adjust as needed:** Track your workouts, progress, and how you feel physically and mentally. Adjust your exercise routine as needed based on your goals, feedback from your body, and any changes in your fitness level or schedule.

### *Sample Exercise Routine for Women Over 50*

This is just an example of the starting steps on your intermittent fasting combined with exercise on the 14:10 fasting schedule. Once you feel comfortable with your level of fitness and your fasting times, you can add more time to the exercises or change them completely. Remember, this is about your journey. Keep the points above in mind when making your schedule, and you'll be good to go!

This sample includes a mix of cardiovascular, strength training, flexibility, and balance exercises to promote overall health and well-being:

| | Monday | Tuesday | Wednesday | Thursday | Friday | Saturday | Sunday |
|---|---|---|---|---|---|---|---|
| **Morning:** | Eating window | Eating window | Eating window | Eating window | Eating window | Eating window | Eating window |
| **9–11 a.m.** | 30 min. yoga | Rest day | 30 min. Swim | Rest day | Any day | Rest day | 30 min. walk |
| **Noon:** | Eating window | Eating window | Eating window | Eating window | Eating window | Eating window | Eating window |
| **12–4 p.m.** | 30 min. Tai Chi | Rest day | 30 min. Wall Pilates | Rest day | Any day | Rest day | 30 min. yoga |

| Evening: | Eating window | Eating window | Eating window | Eating window | Eating window | Eating window | Eating window |
|---|---|---|---|---|---|---|---|
| 5–7 p.m. | 30 min. Swim | Rest day | 30 min. Tai Chi | Rest day | Any day | Rest day | 30 min. Wall Pilates |
| Night: | Fast | Fast | Fast | Fast | Fast | Fast | Fast |
| 8 p.m.–8 a.m. | Relax/ sleep | Relax/ sleep | Relax/ sleep | Relax/ sleep | Relax/ sleep | Relax/ sleep | Relax/ sleep |

Feel free to modify this routine based on your fitness level, preferences, and schedule. Remember to listen to your body, take rest days as needed, and adjust the intensity and duration of your workouts accordingly.

Keep track of your workouts, progress, and physical and mental feelings. Use a fitness journal, smartphone app, or wearable fitness tracker to monitor your activity levels, heart rate, and calories burned. Pay attention to how your body responds to different types of exercise, timings, and intensities, and adjust your routine as needed to optimize results and prevent burnout or injury.

As you continue your fitness journey, remember that consistency is critical, and small, incremental changes over time can significantly improve your health and well-being. Celebrate your progress, stay committed to your goals, and enjoy the many benefits of regular exercise and intermittent fasting.

In this chapter, we've explored the vital role of exercise in enhancing the effectiveness of intermittent fasting. Whether you prefer walking, swimming, yoga, or strength training, find activities you enjoy and incorporate them into your intermittent fasting lifestyle.

In the next chapter, we'll dive deeper into the nuances of fasting methods to help you maximize the benefits of intermittent fasting and find the method that is best suited for you. Keep up the enthusiasm and dedication as you continue your journey toward a healthier, happier you!

# Help Others See Their 50s as a Time for Transformation

*"Recognizing that you are not where you want to be is a starting point to begin changing your life."*

Deborah Day

You're halfway through your reading journey, which makes this the perfect time to pause and think about a question that encompasses not only your hormonal health but your entire outlook on life. Have you heard about the growth mindset? This concept, developed by psychologist and Stanford professor, Carol Dweck, is a way of viewing the world as a constant opportunity for growth. One of its most powerful tenets is the idea that struggles are the very best opportunities for change. That is, when things are easy, you can progress more or less steadily. But the big spikes in your journey, those that mark "before and after" moments in your life, come from taking something difficult and turning it into something amazing.

At the start of this book, we mentioned that many of the symptoms of hormonal imbalances—including hot flashes, mood swings, poor sleep, and fatigue—can be vastly reduced by intermittent fasting. If you've already commenced your fasting journey, however, then know that you are doing so much more for your body than reducing the impact of menopause. You are building an arsenal that will protect you against Type 2 diabetes, boost your resistance to stress, and help improve your blood pressure and your cholesterol and triglyceride levels. And what about the big energy boost you feel when you wake up? If intermittent fasting is already making a big difference in your quality of life, I hope you can let other women know how you feel.

**By leaving a review on Amazon, you'll let other women in their 50s and beyond where they can find a book on intermittent fasting that is specifically catered to their needs.**

Thanks for helping me spread the word. I hope you enjoy the rest of your reading journey… let's get those advanced fasting strategies in motion!

FIVE

# Advanced Fasting Methods

I ntermittent fasting (IF) has gained widespread popularity for its effectiveness in promoting weight loss, improving metabolic health, and enhancing overall well-being. However, adhering to a one-size-fits-all approach to intermittent fasting can be challenging and unsustainable in the long run. This chapter will delve into the various intermittent fasting methods and discuss how to personalize them to fit your lifestyle and needs. Understanding the different fasting protocols and tailoring them to your preferences can increase the likelihood of long-term success and help you achieve your health and wellness goals.

Broadening Your Understanding of Intermittent Fasting

Before we explore the different intermittent fasting methods, it's essential to understand why a personalized approach is crucial for success. While intermittent fasting can be effective for many individuals, a one-size-fits-all approach to intermittent fasting often fails because it overlooks individuals' diverse needs and preferences. Factors such as age, gender, metabolism, activity level, and dietary preferences all play a role in determining the most suitable fasting method for each person. What works well for one individual may not be sustainable or ideal for another. Personalizing your fasting schedule and approach can ensure long-term commitment and success in achieving your health and wellness goals.

Statistics highlight the importance of personalized fasting methods in ensuring long-term commitment and success. For example, research published in Obesity Reviews indicates that adherence to intermittent fasting regimens tends to decline over time, with many individuals struggling to maintain strict fasting protocols. Additionally, a study published in JAMA Internal Medicine found that while intermittent fasting can lead to significant short-term weight loss, adherence rates drop over the long term, leading to weight regain in many cases.

Personalized fasting methods consider factors such as lifestyle, preferences, and health goals to create sustainable and enjoyable fasting regimens, increasing the likelihood of long-term adherence and success.

## Different Methods of Intermittent Fasting

Intermittent fasting encompasses a variety of fasting protocols, each with its unique principles, benefits, and challenges. Let's explore some of the most popular methods of intermittent fasting:

### *The Time-Related Methods*

### The 12:12 Method

This intermittent fasting schedule is the safest of them all. It gives you a wide window of a food-focused lifestyle while maintaining your fast for health reasons. You have a 12-hour fasting period and a 12-hour eating window. It's that simple! Whatever your reason, the 12:12 method is easy to follow and gives your body a head start on the later, more restrictive, time-based fasting schedules.

*Pros:*

1. Ease of implementation: The 12:12 method is straightforward, making it easy to incorporate into your daily routine.
2. Suitable for individuals new to fasting or concerned about more extended fasting periods.
3. The 12:12 method offers flexibility in meal timing, allowing individuals to adjust their fasting and eating windows to fit their schedules and preferences.

*Cons:*

1. Compared to longer fasting periods, such as 16:8 or 18:6, the 12:12 method may offer fewer metabolic and weight loss benefits, as the fasting window is relatively short.
2. Some individuals may compensate for the fasting period by overeating during the eating window, which can offset any potential benefits of intermittent fasting and hinder weight management efforts.

**The 14:10 Method**

You have a 14-hour fasting period and a 10-hour eating window. Fourteen hours is still a reasonable amount of fasting duration, mainly if you schedule your fasting periods around bedtime and early evening or early morning, depending on your lifestyle. You fast for 14 hours with a ten-hour eating window, giving you plenty of time to eat well-balanced meals and stay hydrated during the fast.

*Pros*:

1. The 14:10 method can be a gentle, more gradual approach to fasting, making it easier to adopt.
2. The 14:10 method offers flexibility in meal timing, allowing individuals to adjust the fasting and eating windows to fit their schedules and preferences.

*Cons:*

1. Some individuals may compensate for the fasting period by overeating during the eating window, which can offset any potential benefits of intermittent fasting and hinder weight management efforts.

**16/8 Method**

The 16/8 method involves fasting for 16 hours and restricting eating to an 8-hour window. This approach is one of the most straightforward forms of intermittent fasting and can be easily integrated into daily life. During fasting, you abstain from consuming calories, allowing your body to enter a state of fat-burning and metabolic rest. Eating is confined to a specific window, typically from noon to 8 pm. However, the timing can be adjusted to suit individual preferences and schedules.

*Pros:*

- Simple and easy to follow
- Flexible eating window
- It can promote weight loss and improve metabolic health

*Cons:*

- It may be challenging for those accustomed to regular snacking
- Requires discipline and consistency

## The Flipped 16:8 Diet, the 8:16

On the flip side, after you feel comfortable and healthy after the traditional 16:8 and its precursors, you could try fasting for 8 hours only but fill your 16-hour eating window with low-calorie snacks throughout the day. A 16-hour eating period will help if you have low blood sugar because you eat more often than the other methods, giving you various foods. Be careful with the 8:16 method, though: It's easy to over-eat when you eat more often, so low-calorie snacks are the way to go. For this method, preparing your snacks beforehand is an excellent way to prevent picking because you are used to larger meals and offsetting your health transformation.

*Pros*

1. By restricting eating to a shorter window, women may consume fewer calories, leading to weight loss.
2. The flipped 16:8 diet's structure is straightforward and easy to follow, making it accessible for women who want to adopt a fasting lifestyle.
3. The fasting window can be tailored to fit individual schedules and preferences, allowing for flexibility in meal timing.

*Cons:*

1. Restricting food intake to a shorter time frame may make consuming an adequate amount of essential nutrients challenging.
2. May interfere with social gatherings or mealtimes with family and friends,

### *Alternate-Day Fasting*

Alternate-day fasting involves fasting every other day, with some versions allowing for limited caloric intake (around 500 calories) on fasting days.

### 5:2 Method

The 5:2 method involves eating normally five days a week and limiting caloric intake to around 500-600 calories on two non-consecutive days. Individuals typically consume low-calorie, nutrient-dense foods such as vegetables, lean protein, and healthy fats on fasting days. This approach allows for greater flexibility and variety in food choices while promoting weight loss and other health benefits associated with intermittent fasting.

*Pros:*

- Allows for flexibility in food choices
- It can promote weight loss and improve metabolic health.
- Provides a structured approach to intermittent fasting

*Cons:*

- Requires calorie counting and meal planning on fasting days
- It may be challenging to adhere to on fasting days
- It may not be suitable for individuals with certain medical conditions or dietary restrictions

**Eat-Stop-Eat**

The Eat-Stop-Eat method involves a 24-hour fast once or twice a week, during which you abstain from consuming calories. This approach allows for complete rest and rejuvenation of the digestive system, promoting fat-burning, autophagy, and other metabolic processes. Fasting days are typically followed by days of normal eating, allowing for greater flexibility and enjoyment of food.

*Pros:*

- Promotes fat-burning and metabolic health
- Allows for complete rest and rejuvenation of the digestive system
- Provides flexibility in fasting frequency and timing

*Cons:*

- Requires discipline and commitment to fasting for 24 hours
- It may be challenging for individuals accustomed to regular meals
- It may not be suitable for individuals with certain medical conditions or dietary restrictions

**OMAD (One Meal A Day)**

The OMAD method involves consuming all daily calories within a single meal and fasting for 23 hours. This approach allows for extended periods of fasting, promoting fat-burning, autophagy, and other metabolic processes. OMAD can be an effective strategy for weight loss, improving metabolic health, and simplifying meal planning and preparation.

*Pros:*

- Simplifies meal planning and preparation
- Promotes fat-burning and metabolic health
- Allows for extended periods of fasting

*Cons:*

- Requires consuming all daily calories within a single meal
- It may be challenging for individuals accustomed to regular meals
- It may not be suitable for individuals with certain medical conditions or dietary restrictions

**Warrior Diet**

The Warrior Diet involves fasting for 20 hours and eating one large meal in a 4-hour eating window. This approach mimics the eating patterns of ancient warriors, who would fast during the day and feast at night. The Warrior Diet promotes fat burning, mental clarity, and overall well-being while still allowing for the enjoyment of food and social gatherings.

*Pros:*

- Mimics natural eating patterns
- Promotes fat-burning and metabolic health
- Allows for enjoyment of food and social gatherings

*Cons:*

- Requires fasting for 20 hours per day
- It may be challenging to adhere to initially
- It may not be suitable for individuals with certain medical conditions or dietary restrictions

**Crescendo Fasting**

Crescendo fasting starts with a shorter fast and gradually builds up to more extended fasting periods. This approach is ideal for beginners or those new to intermittent fasting, as it allows for a gradual transition and adaptation to fasting. Crescendo fasting can be customized to fit individual preferences and goals, providing a flexible and sustainable approach to intermittent fasting.

*Pros:*

- Gradual transition and adaptation to fasting
- Allows for customization based on individual preferences and goals
- A sustainable approach to intermittent fasting

*Cons:*

- It may require patience and perseverance as fasting periods increase
- Requires careful monitoring of hunger levels and energy levels
- It may not be suitable for individuals with certain medical conditions or dietary restrictions

## Personalizing Your Fasting Schedule

Now that we've explored the different intermittent fasting methods, it's time to personalize your fasting schedule to fit your lifestyle and needs. The effectiveness of your fasting schedule relies on your ability to be consistent and honest with your reasons for fasting, your goals, and your planning skills. Planning your fasting around your schedule can be broken down into levels, regardless of your preferred type.

**Level one schedule—eat anytime:** With the first schedule, your day is entirely up to you. You can eat within your eating window, depending on the type (12-hour eating time window to 4-hour warrior window, etc.), whenever you want and have the time. For example, your eating window is from 8 a.m. to 8 p.m., but if you call at 8:05 a.m., eating at 9:00 a.m. or 12 p.m. is also acceptable.

**Level two schedule—hungry window:** Most of us eat when hungry and bored. By only eating when hungry, limiting the food you have while bored, and staying within your eating window, the chances of overeating are slim. If your eating window is from 8 a.m. to 6 p.m., but you aren't hungry at 8 a.m., skipping your next meal (lunch, in this case, if you have three meals a day) will give you more time to focus on exercise and self-improvement.

**Level three schedule—delayed hunger:** When you get hungry within your eating window, wait an hour to eat. If the hour passes your eating window, skip that meal or dish. However, if this meal goes past your eating window, you don't start the eating period later the following day; instead, skip that meal entirely. For example, if your eating window is from 10 am–6 pm, you can (if allowed) eat breakfast at work at 11 am. If you aren't hungry at 6 pm (when your eating period ends) because you worked in the garden and would instead take a shower than a meal, skip dinner and have breakfast.

**Level four schedule—time-sensitive meals:** This level is slightly more restricted than the others. For it to work, you must eat at certain times within your eating window and only at those times. If you practice alternate-day fasting, this schedule should be on a fast day, not a typical day. If you choose 16:8 for your fasting day, your eating window could be 10 am–6 pm. In this case, you will have to eat breakfast at 10–10:05 am and dinner at 5–5:05 pm or skip these meals entirely (unless you will skip both) if you are busy during these times. This isn't a means to punish you for not paying attention to the time. Think of it as an incentive to stick to a schedule you created for your benefit.

**Level five schedule—half a window:** At level five, the practicality of your schedule plays a role. You eat half of what you would have eaten in your eating window: This is the key to helping your fasting synergize with your lifestyle and routine by practicing portion control and meal planning for the next day. If you eat half of what you usually eat, you most likely have a calorie deficit. This will help with weight loss and means you have more time during the day (or night) to do what you love.

**Level six schedule:** You eat half of what you would have eaten within your eating window but only at specific times. Level six combines level five and level four. This is the most practical type of scheduling with intermittent fasting because you save time in food prep for the following day, opening up your schedule, and the smaller portions of food will help you lose weight and decrease sugar spikes, which interfere with your hormones.

Intermittent fasting is only as effective as your schedule and routine commitment. Still, we don't live on our own island (if only!). Our working and sleeping habits interfere with our lifestyle goals. We must time our fasting and exercise schedules around working and personal hours for sleep and spending time with family and on ourselves. One of the benefits of intermittent fasting compared to diets is we don't obsess about food, but that doesn't mean we treat mealtimes as second-fiddle to our commitments.

Our work schedules and sleeping patterns remain the same, and we may be unable to skip the monthly dinner at Fran's house. Still, we can use this to our advantage when planning our schedules. If you work (or work from home) from 8–5, you could choose one of the time-related methods that will work the best for your work schedule, or if you must be in bed by 8 pm because your shift starts at 5 am, the crescendo might work for you because it's more flexible.

Please find printable templates below for each type of fasting method.

The key is:

**Eating window**: E.W.

**Fasting window:** Blank space (you can use the blank spaces to write notes about your diet, feelings, and progression).

**Each eating period begins and ends with Meal:** Feel free to write the meal or snack you had at that time for record keeping.

*The Time Related Method/s:*

|        | 12:12                       | 14:10          | 16:8 | 8:16           |
|--------|-----------------------------|----------------|------|----------------|
| 4 a.m. |                             |                |      |                |
| 5 a.m. |                             |                |      |                |
| 6 a.m. |                             |                |      |                |
| 7 a.m. |                             |                |      | E.W.<br><br>Meal: |
| 8 a.m. | Eating window.<br>(E.W)<br><br>Meal: |                |      | E.W.           |
| 9 a.m. | E.W.                        | E.W.<br><br>Meal: |      | E.W.           |

| | | | | |
|---|---|---|---|---|
| **9 a.m.** | E.W. | E.W.<br><br>Meal: | | E.W. |
| **10 a.m.** | E.W. | E.W. | | E.W. |
| **11 a.m.** | E.W. | E.W. | E.W.<br><br>Meal: | E.W. |
| **12 p.m.** | E.W. | E.W. | E.W. | E.W. |
| **1 p.m.** | E.W.<br><br>Meal: | E.W.<br><br>Meal: | E.W. | E.W.<br><br>Meal: |
| **2 p.m.** | E.W. | E.W. | E.W. | E.W. |
| **3 p.m.** | E.W. | E.W. | E.W. | E.W. |

## *Alternate-Day Fasting:*

| | Monday | Tuesday | Wednesday | Thurs-day | Friday | Saturday | Sunday |
|---|---|---|---|---|---|---|---|
| **5 a.m.** | Fast day | Normal/ exercise day | Fast day | Normal/exercise day | Fast day | Normal/exercise day | Fast day |
| **6 a.m.** | | | | | | | |
| **7 a.m.** | | | | | | | |
| **8 a.m.** | | | | | | | |
| **9 a.m.** | | | | | E.W. Meal: | | |
| **10 a.m.** | | | E.W. Meal: | | E.W. | | |
| **11 a.m.** | | | E.W. | | E.W. | | |
| **12 p.m.** | Eating window. (E.W) Meal: | | E.W. | | E.W. | | E.W. Meal: |
| **1 p.m.** | E.W. | | E.W. | | E.W. | | E.W. |
| **2 p.m.** | E.W. | | E.W. | | E.W. | | E.W. |
| **3 p.m.** | E.W. | | E.W. | | E.W. | | E.W. |

| | | | | | | | |
|---|---|---|---|---|---|---|---|
| **4 p.m.** | E.W. | | E.W. | | E.W. | | E.W. |
| **5 p.m.** | E.W. | | E.W. | | E.W. | | E.W. |
| **6 p.m.** | E.W. | | E.W. | | E.W. | | E.W. |
| **7 p.m.** | E.W. Meal: | | E.W. Meal: | | E.W. | | E.W. Meal: |
| **8 p.m.** | | | | | E.W. | | |
| **9 p.m.** | | | | | E.W. | | |
| **10 p.m.** | | | | | | | |

## Crescendo Fasting:

| | Monday | Tuesday | Wednesday | Thursday | Friday | Saturday | Sunday |
|---|---|---|---|---|---|---|---|
| **4 a.m.** | Normal/ exercise day | Fasting day | Anything day | Fasting day | Anything day | Normal/ exercise day | Fasting day |
| **5 a.m.** | | | | | | | |
| **6 a.m.** | | | | | | | |
| **7 a.m.** | | | | | | | |
| **8 a.m.** | | Eating window. (E.W). | | | | | E.W. Meal: |

| | | Meal: | | | | | |
|---|---|---|---|---|---|---|---|
| 9 a.m. | | E.W. | | | | | E.W. |
| 10 a.m. | | E.W. | | | | | E.W. |
| 11 a.m. | | E.W. | | E.W. Meal: | | | E.W. |
| 12 p.m. | | E.W. | | E.W. | | | E.W. |
| 1 p.m. | | E.W. | | E.W. | | | E.W. |
| 2 p.m. | | E.W. | | E.W. | | | E.W. |
| 3 p.m. | | E.W. | | E.W. | | | E.W. |
| 4 p.m. | | E.W. | | E.W. | | | E.W. |
| 5 p.m. | | E.W. | | E.W. | | | E.W. |
| 6 p.m. | | E.W. | | E.W. Meal: | | | E.W. |
| 7 p.m. | | E.W. Meal: | | | | | E.W. Meal: |
| 8 p.m. | | | | | | | |
| 9 p.m. | | | | | | | |

## *The Eat-Stop-Eat Diet:*

|  | Monday | Tuesday | Wednesday | Thursday | Friday | Saturday | Sunday |
|---|---|---|---|---|---|---|---|
| **4 a.m.** | Fast day | Normal/exercise day | Fast day | Normal/exercise day | Fast day | Normal/exercise day | Fast day |
| **3 p.m.** | | | | | | | |
| **4 p.m.** | | | | | | | |
| **5 p.m.** | | | | | | | |
| **6 p.m.** | Eating window. (E.W). Meal: | | E.W. Meal: | | | | E.W. Meal: |
| **7 p.m.** | | | | | | | |
| **8 p.m.** | | | | | E.W. Meal: | | |
| **9 p.m.** | | | | | | | |
| **10 p.m.** | | | | | | | |

## *The Warrior Diet:* Every day is a fast day.

|  | Monday | Tuesday | Wednesday | Thursday | Friday | Saturday | Sunday |
|---|---|---|---|---|---|---|---|
| **4 p.m.** |  |  |  |  |  |  |  |
| **5 p.m.** | Eating window. (E.W) Meal: | E.W. Meal: |  |  |  |  | E.W. Meal: |
| **6 p.m.** | E.W. | E.W. | E.W. Meal: | E.W. Meal: |  |  | E.W. |
| **7 p.m.** | E.W. | E.W. | E.W. | E.W. | E.W. Meal: | E.W. Meal: | E.W. |
| **8 p.m.** | E.W. (or) | E.W. (or) | E.W. | E.W. | E.W. | E.W. | E.W. |
| **9 p.m.** |  |  | E.W. | E.W. | E.W. | E.W. |  |
| **10 p.m.** |  |  | E.W. (or) | E.W. (or) | E.W. | E.W. |  |
| **11 p.m.** |  |  |  |  | E.W. (or) | E. W. (or) |  |
| **12 p.m.** |  |  |  |  |  |  |  |

## *The OMAD Diet:* Every day is a fast day.

|  | Monday | Tuesday | Wednesday | Thursday | Friday | Saturday | Sunday |
|---|---|---|---|---|---|---|---|
| **9 a.m.** |  |  |  |  |  |  |  |
| **10 a.m.** | Eating window. (E.W) Meal: (or) |  |  |  |  |  |  |
| **11 a.m.** |  |  |  |  |  |  |  |
| **12 p.m.** |  |  | E.W. Meal: (or) |  |  |  |  |
| **1 p.m.** |  |  |  |  |  |  |  |
| **2 p.m.** |  |  |  |  | E.W. Meal: (or) |  |  |
| **3 p.m.** |  |  |  |  |  |  |  |
| **4 p.m.** |  |  |  |  |  |  | E.W. Meal: (or) |
| **5 p.m.** |  |  |  |  |  |  |  |
| **6 p.m.** |  |  |  |  | E.W. Meal: (or) |  |  |
| **7 p.m.** |  |  | E.W. Meal: (or) |  |  |  |  |

| 8 p.m. | E.W. Meal: (or) | | | | | | |
|---|---|---|---|---|---|---|---|
| 9 p.m. | Etc. | | | | | | |
| 10 p.m. | | | | | | | |

Here are some practical steps to help you adopt a fasting schedule that works for you:

1. **Assess your daily routine:** Take stock of your work hours, sleep patterns, family commitments, and other personal obligations. Identify windows of time where fasting would be most feasible and least disruptive to your daily routine.

2. **Choose a fasting method:** Consider the earlier methods and choose one that aligns with your goals, preferences, and lifestyle. Experiment with different methods to find the one that works best for you.

3. **Plan your fasting schedule:** Use worksheets or downloadable templates to map out your weekly fasting schedule. Determine your fasting and eating windows, and plan your meals accordingly to ensure you meet your nutritional needs.

4. **Be flexible and adaptable**: Remember that intermittent fasting is not about rigid rules or protocols. Be willing to adjust your fasting schedule based on changes in your routine, hunger, and energy levels.

5. **Listen to your body**. Learn how your body responds to fasting and adjust your schedule accordingly. If you feel excessively hungry or tired, consider shortening your fasting window or adding a small snack to your eating window.

## How to Choose What's Best for Your Lifestyle

Choosing the proper fasting method for your lifestyle involves considering several critical factors, including your activity level, work commitments, family responsibilities, and dietary preferences. Here are some questions to help you identify the best fasting method for you:

1. What is your activity level? Consider how your fasting schedule will impact your energy levels and performance during physical activity. Choose a fasting method that allows you to maintain your energy levels and performance throughout the day.
2. What are your work commitments? Consider your work schedule and how fasting will fit into your daily routine. Choose a fasting method that aligns with your work hours and allows you to remain focused and productive throughout the day.
3. What are your family responsibilities? Consider how fasting will affect your family meals and social gatherings. Choose a fasting method that allows you to enjoy meals with your family and participate in social events without feeling deprived or restricted.
4. What are your dietary preferences? When choosing a fasting method, consider your food preferences and

dietary restrictions. Choose a method that allows you to enjoy a variety of foods while still meeting your nutritional needs.

5. How flexible are you? Consider how flexible and adaptable you are to changes in your routine and eating habits. Choose a fasting method that fits seamlessly into your lifestyle and allows for adjustments.

Don't let a rigid diet and exercise routine remove the joy of living in the now! Flexibility is crucial to your success in work and relationships. Your intermittent fasting diet shouldn't be any different! Here is a quick questionnaire that can give you some guidance on picking a fasting method:

You can print it or use a pencil to select the option.

| Why did you choose intermittent fasting? | |
|---|---|
| To eat on a schedule. | 1 |
| To go on a diet that lets me have normal days. | 2 |
| To control my hormones and weight. | 3 |
| To control my eating. | 4 |
| To have an excuse to eat for hours. | 5 |

| How often do you forget to eat or miss meals because of time? | |
|---|---|
| Every day. | 1 |
| A few times a week. | 2 |
| One week, every day. The next week, not often. | 3 |
| Not very often. | 4 |
| I normally remember to eat at night. | 5 |
| **How often do you want to exercise?** | |
| Everyday. | 1 |
| Three times a week. | 2 |
| Twice a week. | 3 |
| Once a week. | 4 |
| Once a month. | 5 |
| **How many diets have you been on in the past?** | |
| None. | 1 |
| A few, none of them worked. | 2 |

| A few, some of them worked. | 3 |
| Lots, some worked, some didn't. | 4 |
| Don't mention the word diet to me. | 5 |

| **Do you suffer from any illness currently, or have in the past?** |
| No. |
| Yes, I have diabetes. |
| Yes, I have cardiac and circulation issues. |
| Yes, there is a family history of cardiac or circulation issues. |
| Yes, I have cancer. |
| Yes, I had cancer, but I'm in remission. |
| Yes, I have hypertension or suffered from it in the past. |
| Yes, I have anorexia or bulimia nervosa or suffered from it in the past. |

This chapter explored the different intermittent fasting methods and discussed how to personalize them to fit your lifestyle and needs. You can choose the best approach by understanding the principles and benefits of each fasting method and considering key factors such as activity level, work commitments, and dietary preferences. Whether you prefer the simplicity of the 16/8 method, the flexibility of the 5:2 method, or the gradual progression of crescendo fasting, there is a fasting method that can fit seamlessly into your lifestyle and help you achieve your health and wellness goals.

In the next chapter, we'll address some common challenges and obstacles you may encounter on your intermittent fasting journey—and provide practical solutions to keep you on track. Keep up the enthusiasm and dedication as you continue to personalize your intermittent fasting journey and reap its many benefits!

SIX

# Navigating Challenges

*"Success is stumbling from failure to failure with no loss of enthusiasm."*

Winston S. Churchill

I ntermittent fasting is a journey filled with ups and downs, triumphs and setbacks. But remember, every stumble is an opportunity to learn and grow. In this chapter, we'll explore some of the common challenges you might encounter along your intermittent fasting journey and provide you with practical strategies for overcoming them. With the right tools and mindset, you can confidently navigate these obstacles and continue moving toward your health and wellness goals.

## Common Obstacles

Embarking on an intermittent fasting journey can face its fair share of challenges. From dealing with hunger pangs to managing social pressures and combating fatigue, it's essential to be prepared for the hurdles that may arise. Here are some common obstacles you might encounter and actionable advice for overcoming them:

**Hunger Pangs**

Feeling hungry during fasting periods is a shared experience, especially in the initial weeks of starting fasting. However, as our bodies adapt to the change, the intensity of hunger tends to diminish over time. While adjusting and managing hunger and cravings can be challenging, there are effective strategies to help.

Focusing on hydration is critical to curbing hunger and cravings. Water fills our stomachs, making it harder to overeat, and it also plays a crucial role in regulating hunger and thirst signals. Drinking plenty of water throughout the day aids in processing food and nutrients, providing a pathway for digestion.

During eating windows, incorporating snacks and meals rich in protein can help control hunger. Protein supports hormone regulation and aids digestion, helping keep hunger at bay. Additionally, prioritizing vegetables, which are high in fiber, can prolong the feeling of fullness and satiety. Fiber-rich foods aid digestion and nutrient absorption, creating a sense of satisfaction and reducing the urge to eat frequently. Over time, as our bodies adapt to the fasting regimen, hunger pangs become less intense, making it easier to stick to the fasting schedule and achieve our health goals.

**Social Pressures**

Dining out with friends or attending social gatherings can present challenges when following an intermittent fasting protocol. Friends, family, and societal norms often dictate mealtimes and eating habits, leading to feelings of isolation or judgment when fasting during social gatherings. Additionally, well-meaning but unsolicited advice from others may undermine confidence and commitment to fasting goals.

Communicating openly and confidently about personal health choices while intermittent fasting is essential for overcoming social pressure. Finding like-minded individuals or joining online communities dedicated to intermittent fasting can provide a sense of belonging and support. Sharing experiences, tips, and encouragement with others facing similar challenges can boost motivation and confidence in fasting practices.

Also, remember to practice mindfulness and self-compassion in navigating social pressure. Recognizing that occasional lapses or deviations from fasting schedules are normal and reframing setbacks as learning opportunities rather than failures can help maintain resilience and long-term commitment to intermittent fasting goals.

**Loss of Energy**

Some people may experience fatigue or low energy levels, especially when starting intermittent fasting. Your concentration and energy levels are tied to your diet. The food you eat gives your body energy. As the body adjusts to changes in eating patterns, fluctuations in blood sugar levels and nutrient intake can lead to feelings of fatigue and lethargy, particularly during fasting periods. This can impact daily activities, productivity, and overall well-being.

During eating windows, it's essential to prioritize nutrient-dense foods. Incorporating lean proteins, carbohydrates, healthy fats, and plenty of fruits and vegetables can sustain energy levels throughout the day. Additionally, opting for smaller, more frequent meals during eating windows can help stabilize blood sugar levels and prevent energy crashes.

Hydration is also crucial in combating fatigue while fasting. Drinking plenty of water throughout the day helps maintain hydration levels. It supports metabolic function, which can alleviate feelings of sluggishness.

Strategic meal timing can further optimize energy levels during intermittent fasting. Consuming larger meals closer to the beginning or end of eating windows when energy needs are highest can help sustain energy levels throughout fasting periods.

Finally, prioritizing adequate rest and stress management techniques, such as meditation or gentle exercise, can support overall energy levels and resilience while practicing intermittent fasting. By addressing these factors, women over 50 can effectively manage energy loss and thrive on their fasting journey.

**Bad Breath**

Fasting causes our mouths to lack moisture, which increases the acetone in our saliva. Acetone is present in your breath while fasting because it accelerates the fat-burning process. Dehydration is also a cause of bad breath, so the combination of the lack of moisture and dehydration could create an unpleasant situation for your mouth and affect the taste of your next meal.

Good oral hygiene is the number one way to combat bad breath. Compared to the other obstacles, oral hygiene is relatively easy to combat. A good fluoride toothpaste, alcohol-free mouthwash, and a toothbrush just right for your teeth (soft-hard bristles) are all it takes. Sugar-free gum may also give temporary relief.

## Dealing with Cheat Days

Cheat days happen to the best of us, and they're nothing to feel guilty about. Whether you indulge in your favorite dessert or veer off your fasting schedule, it's essential to approach cheat days with compassion and understanding. Not giving up when you have cheated a day is the key to helping you stay consistent long-term.

Here's how to bounce back from a cheat day:

- **Reframe Your Mindset:** Instead of viewing a cheat day as a setback, consider it an opportunity to indulge and enjoy guilt-free. Remember, in the same way, one day of fasting will change anything; one day of indulgence won't undo all your progress. Re-evaluating why you started will put things in perspective and help clear your mind. Focusing on the positives of your journey and how far you have come is a great way to deal with your guilt about going off-track.

- **Get Back on Track:** Rather than dwelling on your slip-up, focus on getting right back into your fasting routine. It is as simple as that. Fasting is what you do! Start fresh the next day with a healthy, balanced meal and recommit yourself to your routine.

Suppose you have cheat days too often or struggle to get back into your routine. In that case, you may be experiencing burnout. It's essential to reassess your needs and lifestyle to avoid feeling overwhelmed. Utilize the chart in Chapter 5 to identify areas where adjustments can be made. Consider modifying your fasting schedules by trying a different, less intense method and gradually building your way up to find what works best.

Modifying your meals can help sustain your fast while still enjoying the nutritious foods you love. Explore healthy recipes with ingredients that align with your preferences to make fasting more enjoyable and sustainable.

It's also crucial to recognize if you're overworking yourself physically. Taking a few rest days and incorporating less intense workouts can help prevent burnout and allow your body to recover. Gradually build yourself back up to a comfortable activity level, prioritizing self-care and balance in your routine.

Remember, adjusting and making changes along the way is okay to support your overall well-being on your intermittent fasting journey!

## Overcoming Plateaus

Plateaus are common in any weight loss or wellness journey, and intermittent fasting is no exception. A plateau (in this case) is when your weight loss has reached a limit, and you don't see any more progress, regardless of how hard you try. These can be frustrating and might make you think you have reached your limit. You haven't! You are almost there. If you find yourself stuck in a rut and not seeing the progress you'd hoped for, don't despair. Here are some strategies for breaking through a plateau and reigniting your progress:

- **Change Up Your Routine:** If you've been following the same fasting schedule for an extended period, consider switching things up. Try experimenting with different fasting protocols and meal timings or incorporating more and or/ physical activity into your routine. An article By DoFasting Editorial suggests incorporating intermittent fasting variability to break through a plateau. This involves alternating fasting lengths or schedules to prevent the body from adapting to a consistent fasting routine, promoting continued fat loss.
- **Focus on Nutrition:** Reassess your dietary habits and ensure you're fueling your body with nutrient-dense foods that support your health and wellness goals. Pay attention to portion sizes, minimize

processed foods, and prioritize whole, unprocessed foods. Additionally, most people just need to limit their calorie intake. Eating fewer calories creates a deficit, where you burn more calories than you take in. A calorie deficit is a simple equation and a requisite for weight loss. A deficit of 250-500 calories daily is sufficient for most people to lose weight.

## Staying Motivated

Staying motivated throughout the intermittent fasting journey is crucial for long-term success, especially when faced with challenges like hitting a plateau. It's essential to delve deeper into the reasons behind your commitment beyond just wanting to lose weight. Reflecting on how a healthier lifestyle aligns with your goals and aspirations can provide a strong foundation for motivation.

Here are some tips for staying motivated and inspired along the way:

**Setting realistic/achievable goals:** Goal setting is key to staying motivated. Reaching these milestones boosts confidence and encourages further progress. Focus on the positive outcomes of intermittent fasting, emphasizing its longevity and overall well-being benefits. Visualizing a future filled with health and vitality can serve as a powerful motivator, showcasing the potential rewards of your hard work.

Additionally, Break down larger objectives into smaller, more manageable steps to make progress feel attainable. By focusing on gradual improvements and celebrating each milestone, you'll maintain momentum and stay motivated throughout your intermittent fasting journey.

**Having a support system:** First and foremost, a support system, such as a fasting buddy or friend, offers understanding and empathy. They can relate to your struggles, share their experiences, and provide practical advice on overcoming obstacles. Knowing that someone else is going through similar challenges can provide a sense of solidarity and reassurance that you're not alone in your journey.

Moreover, having a fasting buddy or support group creates a sense of accountability. When you have someone to report to or share your progress with, you're more likely to stay committed to your fasting schedule and goals. The fear of letting them down or the desire to share your achievements can be powerful motivators to stick to your plan.

**Celebrate Wins:** Celebrating small and significant victories is essential for maintaining morale. Rewards don't have to be food-related; simple pleasures like a movie night with friends or treating yourself to new gym clothes can serve as meaningful incentives. Whether reaching a fasting milestone, fitting into a pair of jeans, or sticking to your fasting schedule for a week straight, celebrate your progress and use it as motivation to keep going.

In this chapter, we've explored some common challenges you might encounter on your intermittent fasting journey and provided you with practical strategies for overcoming them.

Remember, intermittent fasting is a marathon, not a sprint, and facing obstacles along the way is normal. By approaching challenges with resilience, determination, and a positive mindset, you can navigate any road bumps and continue moving toward your health and wellness goals.

In the next chapter, we'll delve into how to make these changes permanent, transforming your diet and entire lifestyle. Keep up the fantastic work, and remember that you can achieve anything you want!

# SEVEN

## Transforming Your Life

> "*Transformation is not a future event; it's a present-day activity.*"
>
> Jullian Michaels

L et this quote be your guiding light as you embark on the final leg of your transformative journey. In this chapter, we'll focus on sustaining your gains through intermittent Fasting and promoting long-term well-being. Remember, the journey doesn't end with achieving a certain weight or balance; it's a lifestyle change that requires ongoing effort. Let's dive into how you can maintain your achievements and continue thriving on your wellness journey.

## Sustaining Hormonal Balance and Weight

As the previous chapters show, achieving and maintaining hormonal balance is crucial for overall health, well-being, and longevity. Hormones interact intricately, and any imbalance can have significant effects on our health. To sustain hormonal balance and manage weight effectively, we must take an active role in our lifestyle choices.

One of the main hormones affected by lifestyle choices is thyroid hormone, which plays a vital role in metabolism and weight regulation. Hypothyroidism, often experienced by women over 50, can lead to weight gain exacerbated by poor dietary habits and lack of exercise. Conversely, hyperthyroidism can result in weight loss and sleep disturbances. Menopause, characterized by decreased estrogen levels, is another significant hormonal shift experienced by women over 50. While menopause can last several years, intermittent Fasting can provide a sense of control and accomplishment during this transitional phase. Our estrogen levels also play a crucial role in mood, cognition, and physical changes. Lifestyle factors such as fitness level, diet, and sleep quality influence estrogen distribution in the body.

Including whole foods like brown rice and sweet potatoes in an intermittent fasting diet can help stabilize blood sugar levels and promote hormonal balance. In maintaining hormonal balance and weight, it's important to prioritize nutritious foods, regular exercise, and quality sleep. Avoiding sugary and starchy foods can prevent blood sugar spikes and support overall health. Additionally, incorporating mind-body practices like meditation and gratitude exercises can help reduce stress levels and promote hormonal balance.

By making conscious lifestyle choices and embracing intermittent Fasting, women can support their hormonal health and achieve optimal well-being. Remember, the journey to hormonal balance and weight management is ongoing, but with dedication and perseverance, it's achievable. It's time to focus on maintaining that balance to support your long-term success with practical Habits. Incorporate everyday habits into your routine, such as regular exercise, managing stress effectively, prioritizing sleep, and consuming a balanced diet rich in nutrient-dense foods.

Let's prioritize our health and well-being daily, taking small steps towards a vibrant and balanced life.

### Sleep and Stress Management

Sleep and stress management are integral components of maintaining hormonal balance and overall well-being. Here's how you can optimize your sleep and manage stress effectively:

- **Sleep Optimization:** Practice good sleep hygiene by establishing a consistent sleep schedule, creating a relaxing bedtime routine, optimizing your sleep environment, and avoiding caffeine and electronics before bed. Aim for seven to nine hours of sleep per night and establish a consistent sleep schedule to optimize hormone production and regulation. Quality

184 • INTERMITTENT FASTING FOR WOMEN OVER 50 SIMPLIF...

sleep also supports mood, energy levels, and cognitive function.

- **Stress Management**: Chronic stress can disrupt hormonal balance and contribute to weight gain. Incorporate stress-relieving activities into your daily routine, such as mindfulness meditation, deep breathing exercises, yoga, spending time in nature, and engaging in hobbies you enjoy.

## Maintaining Energy Levels

Sustaining energy levels is essential for feeling your best and staying productive throughout the day. Here's how you can maintain optimal energy levels:

- **Intermittent Fasting and Exercise**: Continue practicing intermittent Fasting and incorporating regular exercise into your routine to support sustained energy levels and overall vitality. In fact, a study done in 2020 by Nugraha stated that intermittent Fasting increases energy. When you fast, you have increased concentration because of your body's newly created cells. This signals your brain that your surroundings are safe, and you focus on your thoughts and actions.
- **Proper Hydration:** Stay hydrated by drinking adequate water throughout the day. Dehydration can lead to fatigue and low energy levels. Staying hydrated is also essential for hormone regulation and metabolic function. Drink plenty of water throughout

the day to support digestion, nutrient absorption, and detoxification processes. Limit caffeine and alcohol intake, which can interfere with hydration and hormonal balance.

- **Nutrient-Dense Foods**: Consume a balanced diet consisting of whole, nutrient-dense foods that provide sustained energy, such as fruits, vegetables, lean proteins, whole grains, and healthy fats.

## Emotional and Spiritual Well-being

Emotional and spiritual well-being are equally important components of a balanced and fulfilling life. A balanced emotional and spiritual life contributes to improved mental, emotional, and physical health. Research suggests that spirituality and emotional well-being are closely linked, with benefits ranging from reduced stress and anxiety to enhanced resilience and a greater sense of purpose and meaning in life.

Spirituality can profoundly affect mental health by providing a sense of connection to something greater than oneself, fostering hope and optimism, and offering a framework for coping with life's challenges. Similarly, the 8 dimensions of well-being identified by Colorado State University-Pueblo include spiritual wellness as an integral component of overall health, emphasizing the importance of finding meaning, purpose, and fulfillment in life.

Mind-body practices such as meditation and gratitude exercises are powerful tools for cultivating emotional and spiritual well-being. As explored in articles from Discovery Villages and Circle Square Oval, meditation promotes relaxation, reduces stress, and enhances self-awareness and mindfulness. For fasting women, meditation can be particularly beneficial in managing the stressors of daily life, navigating transitions such as menopause, and fostering a greater sense of peace and balance.

As highlighted by the University of Utah Healthcare and Positive Psychology, gratitude exercises involve intentionally focusing on and appreciating the positive aspects of life. Practicing gratitude has been linked to numerous health benefits, including improved mood, enhanced resilience, and better overall well-being. Incorporating gratitude into daily life can help counteract negative thinking patterns, foster a greater sense of contentment, and promote emotional resilience during challenging times.

Choose a place in your home where you feel the most comfortable and ask yourself soul-searching questions like:

- Why am I doing this (empowering myself through diet and exercise)?
- What are my goals for the future?
- What have I already accomplished?
- How do I acknowledge my achievements?

In addition to these practices, enhancing spiritual health can involve exploring personal beliefs, values, and practices that provide a sense of meaning and purpose. This may include engaging in spiritual practices such as prayer, mindfulness, connection with nature, and participating in community or religious activities that support spiritual growth and connection.

By integrating mind-body practices and cultivating spiritual wellness, women can experience greater emotional resilience, enhanced overall well-being, and a deeper connection to themselves and the world around them. These practices complement the physical benefits of intermittent Fasting, contributing to a holistic approach to health and wellness in midlife and beyond.

## FAQs

You may encounter questions and uncertainties as you continue your intermittent fasting journey. Here are some frequently asked questions and straightforward answers to help guide you:

Can I fast every day?

- Yes, but this depends on the type of fast. If you follow a time-related schedule, fasting every day is safe. If you prefer the OMAD or Stop-Eat-Stop schedule, fasting every day could be unsafe.

Can I fast if I have a chronic illness like type 2 diabetes, hypertension, or other conditions?

- Yes! While Fasting won't cure these illnesses, fasting with chronic diseases may help your state of mind and general well-being. However, it is always best to talk to your healthcare provider first.

Can I still drink alcohol?

- Yes! Alcohol contains a lot of calories, so bear that in mind, but drinking alcohol in your eating window is perfectly fine.

How soon will I see the results?

- You get back what you put in. Depending on your adherence and goals, you can expect to see results in as little as two weeks.

Is intermittent Fasting a diet?

- No. Intermittent Fasting is a lifestyle that incorporates alternative eating schedules to help with weight loss, energy levels, and general well-being.

Is intermittent Fasting a new thing or just a fad?

- No. For thousands of years, various groups have practiced intermittent Fasting to help with longevity and self-control, as well as religiously for spirituality and purpose.

Is it safe to exercise while I'm fasting?

- Yes! Exercise paired with intermittent will only accelerate your progress. Start slow, listen to your body, stay hydrated, and prioritize your safety and well-being above all else.

What can I do if I feel faint during my fast?

- Increase your water intake and rest until you feel better. These feelings are more common at the beginning of the fast, and they will disappear after a few weeks. Drinking something low in calories but electrolytes (like a low-calorie energy drink) is also okay. Additionally, eat nutrient-dense and balanced meals during your fasting window.

What can I drink during my fasting period?

- Anything! Just keep your goals in mind when choosing. If your goal is weight loss, drinking calories might not be the best choice.

Will I lose weight quickly?

- This depends on the fast and the amount of exercise you do. Ultimately, weight loss requires a calorie deficit. Choosing a fasting method with a shorter eating window may help create a bigger deficit, resulting in faster weight loss.

What can I eat during fasting periods?

- During fasting periods, it's essential to abstain from consuming calories. Stick to water, herbal tea, black coffee, and other non-caloric beverages to stay hydrated and curb hunger.

As you've learned, transforming your life is a multifaceted journey. Let's review what we've covered and discuss the next steps in your quest for a balanced, healthy life.

## Share the Good News

I hope this book has made a difference to your quality of life, and your daily enjoyment of it. We have provided you with vital tips on how to get the most from fasting and shared a host of recipes and advanced strategies to boost its efficiency.

If you feel more energetic, confident, and resilient thanks to intermittent fasting, I hope you can pay it forward and let other women know where they can find all the information they need to achieve optimal hormonal balance.

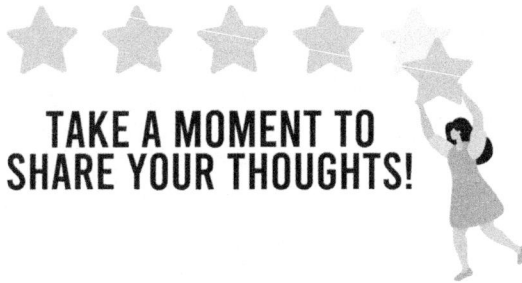

## TAKE A MOMENT TO SHARE YOUR THOUGHTS!

Thanks for your help. Here's to healthy eating, a great night's sleep, and all the energy you need to shine in your professional, personal, and social life.

►►►**Click here to leave a review on Amazon!**

# Conclusion

In closing, the journey you've embarked on through this book has been one of personal growth, empowerment, and self-discovery. You've delved into intermittent fasting, unlocking its potential to revolutionize your health and well-being. As you reflect on the insights gained and the practical tools acquired, remember that the essence of this journey lies not just in the destination but in the daily choices you make to nourish your body, mind, and spirit.

The key takeaway from this book is clear: transformation is not a future event; it's a present-day activity. Each day offers an opportunity to step closer to the vibrant, balanced life you envision. By embracing intermittent fasting as more than a dietary strategy but a lifestyle approach, you've equipped yourself with the knowledge and tools to thrive.

As you move forward, I encourage you to keep the success stories shared in mind. Draw inspiration from those who have walked this path before you, and let their achievements fuel your determination. Remember, you have the potential to achieve remarkable things when you believe in yourself and take consistent action.

Now, armed with knowledge and practical tools, it's time to implement them. Remember, the journey towards a vibrant and balanced life is continuous; make each day count and confidently take the next step. Embrace the challenges, celebrate the victories, and never lose sight of the incredible potential within you. Your journey toward optimal health and well-being starts now.

# References

Aayushi. (2022, October 4). *Intermittent fasting: Put a full stop to your cravings in these 5 ways.* Healthshots. https://www.healthshots.com/healthy-eating/nutrition/5-tips-to-manage-cravings-during-intermittent-fasting/

Adrenocorticotropic hormone (Acth): What it is & function. Cleveland Clinic. https://my.clevelandclinic.org/health/articles/23151-adrenocorticotropic-hormone-acth

*Any success stories for 40+ women?* (2022, June 7). Reddit. https://www.reddit.com/r/intermittentfasting/comments/v6z92j/any_success_stories_for_40_women/

*Are you really hungry? How to your understand hunger cues.* (n.d.). Penn Medicine. https://www.pennmedicine.org/updates/blogs/health-and-wellness/2020/april/how-to-understand-hunger-cues

Arthritis Foundation. (n.d.). *12 Benefits of walking.* Arthritis. 12 benefits of walking. Arthritis.https://www.arthritis.org/health-wellness/healthy-living/physical-activity/walking/12-benefits-of-walking

Bedosky, L. (2022, September 22) *Is it safe to work out if you're fasting?* EverydayHealth. https://www.everydayhealth.com/fitness/should-you-work-out-if-youre-fasting/

Benton, E. (2020, April 27). *It's pretty common to hit a weight-loss plateau while doing intermittent fasting.* Women's Health. https://www.womenshealthmag.com/weight-loss/a32223696/intermittent-fasting-plateau/

Berg, E. (2023, August 31). *Dealing with intermittent fasting fatigue: 5 common causes.* Dr Berg. https://www.drberg.com/blog/the-5-reasons-you-get-tired-on-intermittent-fasting

Bokor, V. (n.d.). *Intermittent fasting and plateau: What do I do wrong?* Wefast. https://www.wefast.care/articles/intermittent-fasting-plateau# Brennan, D. (2021, October 25).

Capritto, A. (2020, November 22). *9 Amazing things exercise can do for you after 50.* Livestrong. https://www.livestrong.com/article/13729514-exercise-benefits-over-50/

Cassata, C. (2019, March 21). *How stress can cause a hormonal imbalance.*

Healthline. https://www.healthline.com/health-news/hormone-imbalances-and-how-to-treat-them

Cassetty, S. (2021, June 28). *What to do after a cheat day*. Nutritionistsam. https://www.samanthacassetty.com/post/what-to-do-after-a-cheat-day

Centers for Disease Control and Prevention. (2023, August 1). *Benefits of physical activity*. Centers for Disease Control and Prevention. https://www.cdc.gov/physicalactivity/basics/pa-health/index.htm

Chevelle, B. (n.d.) .*Weight watchers Mexican chicken breasts*. Food. https://www.food.com/recipe/weight-watchers-mexican-chicken-breasts-155442

*Chocolate peanut butter avocado pudding*. (2014, September 20). Minimalist Baker. https://minimalistbaker.com/chocolate-peanut-butter-avocado-pudding/

Churchill, W. (n.d.) *Winston S. Churchill quotes*. Goodreads. https://www.goodreads.com/quotes/19742-success-is-stumbling-from-failure-to-failure-with-no-loss

Cleveland Clinic. (2021a). *Androgens: Function, measurement and related disorders*. Cleveland Clinic. https://my.clevelandclinic.org/health/articles/22002-androgens

Cleveland Clinic. (2021b). *Cortisol: What it is, function, symptoms & levels*. Cleveland Clinic. https://my.clevelandclinic.org/health/articles/22187-cortisol

Cleveland Clinic. (2021c, December 21). *Parathyroid hormone: What it is, function & levels*. Cleveland Clinic. https://my.clevelandclinic.org/health/articles/22355-parathyroid-hormone Cleveland Clinic. (2022a).

Cleveland Clinic. (2022b). *Luteinizing hormone: Levels, function & testing*. Cleveland Clinic. https://my.clevelandclinic.org/health/body/22255-luteinizing-hormone

Cleveland Clinic. (2022c, February 15). *Prolactin: What it is, function & symptoms*. Cleveland Clinic. https://my.clevelandclinic.org/health/articles/22429-prolactin

Cleveland Clinic. (2022d, February 15). *Thyroid Hormone: What It Is & Function*. Cleveland Clinic. https://my.clevelandclinic.org/health/articles/22391-thyroid-hormone

Cleveland Clinic. (2022e, February 23). *Hormones: What they are, function & types*. Cleveland Clinic. https://my.clevelandclinic.org/health/articles/22464-hormones

Cleveland Clinic. (2022f, March 23). *Dopamine*. Cleveland Clinic. https://my.clevelandclinic.org/health/articles/22581-dopamine

Cleveland Clinic. (2022g, March 27). *Oxytocin: What it is, function & effects*.

Cleveland Clinic. https://my.clevelandclinic.org/health/articles/22618-oxytocin

Cleveland Clinic. (2022h, April 4). *Hormonal imbalance: Causes, symptoms & treatment.* Cleveland Clinic. https://my.clevelandclinic.org/health/diseases/22673-hormonal-imbalance

Cleveland Clinic. (2023, January 23). *Follicle-stimulating hormone (Fsh): What it is & function.* Cleveland Clinic. https://my.clevelandclinic.org/health/articles/24638-follicle-stimulating-hormone-fsh

CookingOnTheSide. (n.d.). *Weight watchers' applesauce-cranberry oatmeal.* Food. https://www.food.com/recipe/weight-watchers-applesauce-cranberry-oatmeal-223535

COOKGIRl. (n.d.). *Veggie delightful sandwich à la subway recipe.* Food. https://www.food.com/recipe/veggie-delightful-sandwich-la-subway-19330

Cross, M. (2021, June 1). *How intermittent fasting can benefit your mental health.* Nutritionist-Resource. https://www.nutritionist-resource.org.uk/memberarticles/how-intermittent-fasting-can-benefit-your-mental-health

Curves. (2020, November 3). *5 reasons women over 50 need to exercise more.* Curves. https://www.curves.com/blog/move/5-reasons-women-over-50-need-to-exercise-more

DeCesaris, L. (2023, January 18). *How intermittent fasting affects women's hormones.* Rupa Health. https://www.rupahealth.com/post/how-intermittent-fasting-affects-womens-hormones

Debb, W, L. (n.d.). *Easy apricot bites recipe.* Food. https://www.food.com/recipe/easy-apricot-bites-395280

Dempsey, B. (n.d.). *This is the absolute best walking workout for people over 50, according to a physical therapist.* Parade. https://parade.com/health/walking-workout-for-people-over-50

Dewey, E. H. (1894). *The true science of living.* Google Books. Henry Bill. https://books.google.je/books?id=a76A0qJX3k0C&source=gbs_navlinks_s

Diana. (2021, January 21). *Top 5 reasons to try a new recipe.* The PKD iDetitian. https://www.thepkddietitian.com/blog/5-reasons-to-try-new-recipe-PKD

Discover *7 surprising health benefits of swimming over 50.* (2023, June 6). Simply Swim UK. https://www.simplyswim.com/blogs/blog/discover-7-surprising-health-benefits-of-swimming-over-50

Do Fasting Editorial. (2023, March 6). *11 ways to stay motivated during intermittent fasting.* DoFasting Blog. https://dofasting.com/blog/fasting-motivation/

Dwynnie. (n.d.). *Easy Bacon-Wrapped Dates*. Food. https://www.food.com/recipe/easy-bacon-wrapped-dates-169050

Eastman, H. (2018, February 8). *3 ways to bounce back strong after a cheat day*. Bodybuilding. https://www.bodybuilding.com/content/3-ways-to-bounce-back-strong-after-a-cheat-day.html

*Exercising when you're over 50: Best practices and routines*. (n.d.). Australian Seniors. https://www.seniors.com.au/funeral-insurance/discover/exercising-over-50

Fauve. (n.d.). *Sausage balls recipe*. Food. https://www.food.com/recipe/sausage-balls-46078

Falk, M. (2021, December 16). *How to start practicing Tai Chi as a beginner*. Shape. https://www.shape.com/fitness/workouts/tai-chi-for-beginners

*Fasting and depression: Does fasting hurt or help?* (2016, October 30). Psych Central. https://psychcentral.com/depression/fasting-and-depression

*Fitness after 50 - Personal training success story*. (2021, October 25). Personal Training, Online Personal Training for Men and Women over 50, Ottawa, Manor Park, Rockcliffe, New Edinburgh. https://www.evertrainlifestyles.com/blog/fitnessafter50-client-showcase-priscillac

*5 health benefits of yoga for women over 50*. (2022, May 16). Viva Fifty! https://www.vivafifty.com/health-benefits-yoga-over-fifty-50-11900/

Fletcher, L. (2022, November 27). *New data on how intermittent fasting affects female hormones*. Applied Health Sciences. https://ahs.uic.edu/kinesiology-nutrition/news/new-data-on-how-intermittent-fasting-affects-female-hormones/

*Food and health safety*. (n.d.). Foodinsight.org; International Food Information Council. https://foodinsight.org/wp-content/uploads/2018/05/2018-FHS-Report-FINAL.pdf

Gayla. J. (n.d.). *Shredded Brussels sprouts with bacon and onions*. Food. https://www.food.com/recipe/shredded-brussels-sprouts-with-bacon-and-onions-193511

Gilson, J. (2018, September 12). *How to create your own workout plan: A guide for beginners*. Whole Life Challenge. https://www.wholelifechallenge.com/how-to-design-your-own-workout-program-a-guide-for-beginners/

Goodreads. *Deborah Day Quotes*. Accessed May 3, 2024. https://www.goodreads.com/author/quotes/1438286.Deborah_Day#:

Grunke, M. (2021, March 11). *Modifying an exercise: When and how*. Survivor Fitness. https://survivorfitness.org/2021/03/11/modifying-an-exercise-when-and-how/

Habtemariam, A. (n.d.). *Hunger signs: How to recognize and interpret body cues*. Verywell Fit. https://www.verywellfit.com/identify-and-understand-hunger-signals-3495870#toc-how-to-recognize-signs-of-hunger

Harvard Health. (2018, December 4). *What's the best exercise plan for me?* HelpGuide.org. https://www.helpguide.org/harvard/whats-the-best-exercise-plan-for-me.htm

Heather. (n.d.). *Chicken and spinach rigatoni casserole recipe*. Food. https://www.food.com/recipe/chicken-and-spinach-rigatoni-casserole-265132

Hiller-Sturmhöfel, S., & Bartke, A. (1998). *The Endocrine System: An Overview*. Alcohol Health and Research World, 22(3), 153–164. https://www.ncbi.nlm.nih.gov/pmc/articles/PMC6761896/

Hofmann Kruse, F. (2019, June 1). *How Barbara lost those stubborn postmenopausal pounds*. Diet Doctor. https://www.dietdoctor.com/how-barbara-lost-those-stubborn-postmenopausal-pounds

*Honey cinnamon peaches*. (2014, June 20). The Skinny Fork. https://theskinnyfork.com/blog/roasted-honey-cinnamon-peaches

*How does food affect your hormones?* (2021, September 6). Marion Gluck. https://www.mariongluckclinic.com/blog/how-does-food-affect-your-hormones.html

*How to start meditating when you're over 50 and not real sure about it*. (2022, February 22). Circle Square Oval. https://circlesquareoval.com/meditation-tips-for-women-over-fifty/

Huizen, J. (n.d.). *Hormonal Imbalance: Symptoms, Causes, and Treatment*. Medical News Today. https://www.medicalnewstoday.com/articles/321486

Ineeta. (2022, October 20). *5 yoga poses for older women: Yoga for women over 50*. MyYogaTeacher. https://myyogateacher.com/articles/yoga-for-women-over-50#

*Intermittent fasting during menopause: What do you need to know?* (n.d.). Menopause Centre. https://www.menopausecentre.com.au/information-centre/articles/intermittent-fasting-during-menopause-what-do-you-need-to-know/

*Intermittent fasting for hormone balance: Pros and cons*. (2022, July 15). Access Medical Labs Blogs. https://accessmedlab.com/blogs/2022/07/15/intermittent-fasting-for-hormone-balance-pros-and-cons/

*Intermittent fasting for menopause: Can it help symptoms?* (2023, May 17). Health & Her. https://healthandher.com/expert-advice/stress-anxiety/intermittent-fasting-menopause/

Jenny, M. (n.d.). *Warm roasted vegetable Farro salad recipe*. Food. https://www.food.com/recipe/warm-roasted-vegetable-farro-salad-526150

Julesong. (n.d.). *Cauliflower popcorn - Roasted cauliflower recipe.* Food. Retrieved February 10, 2024, from https://www.food.com/recipe/cauliflower-popcorn-roasted-cauliflower-115153

Kabula, J. (2021, April 23). *9 Possible intermittent fasting side effects.* Healthline. https://www.healthline.com/nutrition/intermittent-fasting-side-effects#malnutrition

Kate. (2014, April 25). *Roasted strawberry rhubarb and yogurt parfaits.* Cookie and Kate. https://cookieandkate.com/roasted-strawberry-rhubarb-and-yogurt-parfaits/

Katzen. (n.d.). *Millet & quinoa Mediterranean salad recipe.* Food. https://www.food.com/recipe/millet-quinoa-mediterranean-salad-431132]

King, M. (2014, February 21). *3 ingredient banana cups.* My Whole Food Life. https://mywholefoodlife.com/2014/02/21/3-ingredient-banana-cups/

Kitsune. (n.d.). *Cheese bites (totally addictive) Recipe.* Food. https://www.food.com/recipe/cheese-bites-totally-addictive-345344

Lauren. (2020, November 24). *Simple cabbage and eggs.* Oatmeal with a Fork. https://www.oatmealwithafork.com/simply-cabbage-and-eggs/ Line Up

Lizcano, F., & Guzmán, G. (2014). Estrogen deficiency and the origin of obesity during menopause. *BioMed Research International, 2014.* https://doi.org/10.1155/2014/757461

Media. (2023, August 6). *Hormonal quotes.fm.* https://lineupmedia.fm/hormonal-quotes/

Lorrie. (n.d.). *Lemon rosemary salmon recipe.* Food. https://www.food.com/recipe/lemon-rosemary-salmon-317789

Mandabears. (n.d.). *Mediterranean salmon.* Food. https://www.food.com/recipe/mediterranean-salmon-

Mayo Clinic Staff. (n.d.). *Menopause - Symptoms and causes.* Mayo Clinic. https://www.mayoclinic.org/diseases-conditions/menopause/symptoms-causes/syc-20353397

Marg. (n.d.). *Low fat (but tasty!) buttermilk apple bran muffins.* Food. https://www.food.com/recipe/low-fat-but-tasty-buttermilk-apple-bran-muffins-ww-friendly-101631

*Menopause and intermittent fasting - Plus 5 tips for doing it right.* (2019, May 19). Midday. https://midday.health/blog/menopause-and-intermittent-fasting-plus-5-tips-for-doing-it-right/

Meyers, K. (2023, February 14). *8 powerful ways to find encouragement + motivation for fasting.* Zero Longevity. https://zerolongevity.com/blog/motivation-for-fasting/

Mirj2338. (n.d.). *Honey ginger grilled salmon recipe*. Food. https://www.food. com/recipe/honey-ginger-grilled-salmon-13982

Michaels, J. (n.d.). *Jillian Michaels quotes*. Quotefancy. https://quotefancy. com/quote/1508580/Jillian-Michaels-Transformation-isn-t-a-future-event-it-s-a-present-day-activity

*Mood swings and irritability*. (2020, September 2). Women's Health Network. https://www.womenshealthnetwork.com/symptoms/mood-swings/

Morales-Brown, L. (2024, January 24). *Can intermittent fasting cause headaches?* Medical News Today. https://www.medicalnewstoday.com/arti cles/headaches-with-intermittent-fasting#prevention-tips

Morales, T. (n.d.). *Easy black bean soup*. Food. https://www.food.com/recipe/ easy-black-bean-soup-59796

Mosley, B. (n.d.). *10 low-calorie fruit dessert recipes to try!* Guide to Intermittent Fasting. https://guidetointermittentfasting.com/10-low-calorie-fruit-dessert-recipes-try/

*Mozzarella sticks*. (2019). Food. https://www.food.com/recipe/mozzarella-sticks-30977

MS, A. B., CCN. (2020, May 29). *5 intermittent fasting break-fast recipes for every situation!* AutumnElleNutrition. https://www.autumnellenutrition. com/post/5-intermittent-fasting-break-fast-recipes-for-every-situation-travel ing-brunch-at-work

Munuhe, N. (2022, February 23). *Intermittent fasting snacks: 10 plus healthy bites that will help you stay on track*. BetterMe Blog. https://betterme. world/articles/intermittent-fasting-snacks/

Musial, N., Ali, Z., Grbevski, J., Veerakumar, A., & Sharma, P. (2021). *Perimenopause and first-onset mood disorders: A closer look*. FOCUS, 19(3), 330–337. https://doi.org/10.1176/appi.focus.20200041

Nair, P. M. K., & Khawale, P. G. (2016). Role of therapeutic fasting in women's health: An overview. *Journal of Mid-Life Health, 7*(2), 61. https:// doi.org/10.4103/0976-7800.185325

National Institute on Aging. (2021, September 30). *What is menopause?* National Institute on Aging. https://www.nia.nih.gov/health/what-menopause

*Natural healthcare for your female hormones*. (n.d.). Flo Living. https://floliv ing.com/blog/intermittent-fasting

Nelson, S. (2023, May 2). *An introduction to Pilates over 50*. Rest Less. https:// restless.co.uk/health/healthy-body/introduction-to-pilates-over-50/

Nidirect. (2017, October 27). *Malnutrition*. Nidirect. https://www.nidirect.gov. uk/conditions/malnutrition

*Nif's easy cheesy ham and potato frittata.* (n.d.). Food. https://www.food.com/recipe/nifs-easy-cheesy-ham-and-potato-frittata-4-ww-pts-359829

North American Menopause Society. (2019). *Changes in hormone levels, sexual side effects of menopause.* Menopause. https://www.menopause.org/for-women/sexual-health-menopause-online/changes-at-midlife/changes-in-hormone-levels

*Nutrition and impacts on hormone signaling.* (n.d.). The Institute for Functional Medicine. https://www.ifm.org/news-insights/nutrition-impacts-hormone-signaling/

Nutrition for Change. (2020, May 20). *Top 10 foods to restore hormone balance.* Nutrition 4 Change. https://nutrition4change.com/articles/top-10-foods-to-restore-hormone-balance/

Nystul, J. (2021, June 12). *4 reasons why people over 50 should use resistance bands.* One Good Thing by Jillee. https://www.onegoodthingbyjillee.com/exercising-with-resistance-bands/

OB-GYN, M. (n.d.). *Women's hormones: The main culprits for changes in your health?* Moreland obgyn. https://www.morelandobgyn.com/blog/womens-hormones-the-main-culprits-for-changes-in-your-health

Osborn, C. O. (2017, December 18). *Everything you should know about hormonal imbalance.* Healthline Media. https://www.healthline.com/health/hormonal-imbalance

Peacock, K., & Ketvertis, K. M. (2022, August 11). *Menopause.* Nih.gov; StatPearls Publishing. https://www.ncbi.nlm.nih.gov/books/NBK507826/

Peters, H. (2019, June 6). *In training, consistency is the key to your fitness goals.* NIFS. https://www.nifs.org/blog/in-training-consistency-is-the-key-to-your-fitness-goals

Pouliot, H. (n.d.). *How to prevent bad breath while fasting.* SmartMouth. https://smartmouth.com/oral-health/bad-breath/how-to-prevent-bad-breath-while-fasting/

*Psychological benefits of fasting.* WebMD. https://www.webmd.com/diet/psychological-benefits-of-fasting Broccoli quiche recipe. (n.d.). Food. https://www.food.com/recipe/ww-3-pt-weight-watchers-broccoli-quiche-135647

Ranabir, S., & Reetu, K. (2011). Stress and hormones. *Indian Journal of Endocrinology and Metabolism, 15*(1), 18–22. https://doi.org/10.4103/2230-8210.77573

Ryan. (2021, March 25). *Intermittent fasting meal plan.* Ryan and Alex Duo Life. https://www.ryanandalex.com/intermittent-fasting-meal-plan/ Roasted

Phillips, M. C. L. (2019). Fasting as a therapy in neurological disease. *Nutrients*, *11*(10). https://doi.org/10.3390/nu11102501

*7 reasons why swimming is so good for over 50's.* (2020, April 12). Fitness Drum. https://fitnessdrum.com/swimming-for-over-50s/

*7-day intermittent fasting meal plan.* (2022, January 3). Beauty Bites. https://www.beautybites.org/intermittent-fasting-meal-plan/

*19 fruity, chocolate-rich and creamy healthy desserts.* (2020, June 28). Healthline. https://www.healthline.com/health/food-nutrition/healthy-desserts

*32 top intermittent fasting recipes.32 top intermittent fasting recipes.* (n.d.). Food. https://www.food.com/ideas/intermittent-fasting-recipes-6939

Smart Sites. (2022, March 1). *6 tips to help you meditate better in your 50s.* Discovery Village. https://www.discoveryvillages.com/senior-living-blog/6-tips-to-help-you-meditate-better-in-your-50s/

Smith, R. (2004). Let food be thy medicine. *BMJ: British Medical Journal*, 328(7433), 0. https://www.ncbi.nlm.nih.gov/pmc/articles/PMC318470/

Society for Endocrinology. (2019). *You and Your Hormones from the Society for Endocrinology.* Your Hormones. https://www.yourhormones.info/endocrine-conditions/menopause/

Spritzler , F. (2017, February 27). *14 simple ways to break through a weight loss plateau.* Healthline. https://www.healthline.com/nutrition/weight-loss-plateau

Sharma, H. (2022, September 21). *The world record for fasting.* SoMeDocs: Doctors on Social Media. https://doctorsonsocialmedia.com/the-world-record-for-fasting/

Stampfer, M. J., Hu, F. B., Manson, J. E., Rimm, E. B., & Willett, W. C. (2000). Primary prevention of coronary heart disease in women through diet and lifestyle. *New England Journal of Medicine, 343*(1), 16–22.

Stevens, G. (n.d.). *Success stories.* Gin Stephens, Author and Intermittent Faster. https://www.ginstephens.com/success-stories.html

Streit, L. (2023, February 2). *The importance of variety in your diet.* Healthy for Life Meals Fresh & Healthy Meal Plan Delivery. Healthy for Life Meals. https://www.healthyforlifemeals.com/blog/importance-of-variety-in-your-diet

Susrla, S. (2019, July 3). *How to prevent getting hangry during fasting?* Susarla Primary Care. https://susarlapc.com/how-to-prevent-getting-hangry-during-fasting/

*The #1 reason you need consistent exercise.* (2018, June 12). OSR Physical

Therapy. https://www.osrpt.com/2018/06/reason-you-need-consistent-exercise/

*The best easy beef and broccoli stir-fry recipe.* (n.d.). Food. https://www.food.com/recipe/the-best-easy-beef-and-broccoli-stir-fry-99476

*The health benefits of cycling in your 50s.* (2022, June 23). Discovery Village. https://www.discoveryvillages.com/senior-living-blog/the-health-benefits-of-cycling-in-your-50s/

*38 Hippocrates quotes about health, food and medicine.* 38 Hippocrates quotes about health, food and medicine. (n.d.). Wise Owl Quotes. https://wise owlquotes.com/hippocrates/

Thomson, J. (2022, November 15). *Weight loss stories: Women 50+ who have lost over 50 lbs.* The Perfect Workout. https://www.theperfectworkout.com/weight-loss-stories/

*Tips to cycling when you're older.* (n.d.). WebMD. https://www.webmd.com/healthy-aging/tips-cycling-after-50

Trinh, E. (2020, December 29). *10 ways to keep on track with your fitness goals.* Jefit - #1 Gym / Home Workout App. https://www.jefit.com/work out-tips/10-ways-keep-track-fitness-goals

Tunny, G. (n.d.). *Gene Tunney quotes.* BrainyQuote. https://www.brainyquote.com/quotes/gene_tunney_309238

*2018 Food and health safety.* (n.d.). Foodinsight.org; International Food Information Council. https://foodinsight.org/wp-content/uploads/2018/05/2018-FHS-Report-FINAL.p

University of Illinois Chicago. (2022, October 25). *How intermittent fasting affects female hormones: New evidence comes from study of pre- and post-menopausal obese women on the "warrior diet."* Science Daily. https://www.sciencedaily.com/releases/2022/10/221025150257.htm

*Veggie packed cheesy chicken salad (reduced fat) recipe.* (n.d.). Food. https://www.food.com/recipe/veggie-packed-cheesy-chicken-salad-reduced-fat-279361

Vinall , M. (2021, September 1). *Your hormones Maybe the key to getting a solid night's sleep. Here's how.* Healthline. https://www.healthline.com/health/sleep/how-sleep-can-affect-your-hormone-levels#:

*Walking for good health.* (n.d.). Betterhealth. https://www.betterhealth.vic.gov.au/health/healthyliving/walking-for-good-health#

Welch, A. (2012, November 20). *7 tips to sleep better with menopause.* EverydayHealth. https://www.everydayhealth.com/menopause-pictures/tips-to-sleep-better-with-menopause.aspx

Wharton, W., E. Gleason, C., Sandra, O., M. Carlsson, C., & Asthana, S.

(2012). Neurobiological underpinnings of the estrogen - Mood relationship. *Current Psychiatry Reviews,* 8(3), 247–256. https://doi.org/10.2174/157340012800792957

W, J. (n.d.).*Tortilla soup.* Food. https://www.food.com/recipe/weight-watchers-0-point-tortilla-soup-152207

Wonogiri, H. (2023, April 13). *How to prevent stomach disease during fasting in Ramadan.* Hermina Hospitals. https://herminahospitals.com/en/articles/cara-mencegah-penyakit-lambung-selama-berpuasa-di-bulan-ramadhan.html

*Working out while intermittent fasting.* (n.d.). Prospect Medical. https://www.prospectmedical.com/resources/wellness-center/working-out-while-intermittent-fasting

*Why is it harder for women to lose weight after 40?* (2023, December 27). Franciscan Health Alliance. https://www.franciscanhealth.org/community/blog/why-is-it-harder-for-women-to-lose-weight-after-40

Yates, H. (2021, August 9). *Answers to the 10 most asked questions about intermittent fasting.* HEYlifetraining Fitness and Wellness. https:/

WeightoWellness LLC. (n.d.). Cheat Days 101: How to Incorporate Them into Your Diet. https://weightowellnessllc.com/cheat-days-101-how-to-incorporate-them-into-your-diet/

WeFast.Care. (n.d.). Intermittent Fasting Plateau. https://www.wefast.care/articles/intermittent-fasting-plateau#

Anton, S. (n.d.). Intermittent Fasting Plateau. https://drstephenanton.com/intermittent-fasting-plateau/

Women's Health Magazine. (n.d.). How to Break Through an Intermittent Fasting Plateau. https://www.womenshealthmag.com/weight-loss/a32223696/intermittent-fasting-plateau/

DoFasting. (n.d.). Intermittent Fasting Plateau: 8 Tips on How to Break It. https://dofasting.com/blog/intermittent-fasting-plateau/

Healthline. (n.d.). 6 Things to Do When You Hit a Weight-Loss Plateau. https://www.healthline.com/nutrition/weight-loss-plateau

Centers for Disease Control and Prevention (CDC). "Physical Activity and Health." https://www.cdc.gov/physicalactivity/basics/pa-health/index.htm

Curves. "5 Reasons Women Over 50 Need to Exercise More." https://www.curves.com/blog/move/5-reasons-women-over-50-need-to-exercise-more

Livestrong. "Exercise Benefits for Over 50." https://www.livestrong.com/article/13729514-exercise-benefits-over-50/

Cone Health. "4 Benefits of Exercising Over 50." https://www.conehealth.com/services/rehabilitation/4-benefits-of-exercising-over-50/

WebMD. "Slideshow: Exercise After Age 50." https://www.webmd.com/fitness-exercise/ss/slideshow-exercise-after-age-50

Seniors.com.au. "Exercising Over 50." https://www.seniors.com.au/funeral-insurance/discover/exercising-over-50

Foods For Hormone Balance—10 Cortisol Foods To Avoid Today 2024. https://babyjoyjoy.com/foods-for-hormone-balance/

Exploring the Allure of Weight Loss Supplements: A Comprehensive Overview - UdnfesUdnfes. https://udnfes.com/exploring-the-allure-of-weight-loss-supplements-a-comprehensive-overview/

5 Ways to Manage Nutrition Intake While Intermittent Fasting – Level 9 Personal Training. https://level9personaltraining.com/5-ways-to-get-enough-nutrition-while-intermittent-fasting/

What is a Balanced Diet? | Unilever Health | Unilever. https://www.unilever.co.za/brands/health/articles/what-is-a-balanced-diet/

Printed in Great Britain
by Amazon